CTG
Made
Easy

THIRD EDITION

Susan M Gauge BSc (Hons) SRN SCM ADM ONC
Clinical Midwife, Delivery Suite, Birmingham Women's Healthcare NHS Trust

Christine Henderson MA (Warks) MTD DipN (Lond) DPHE RM RN
Senior Research Fellow, School of Health Sciences, The University of Birmingham, UK

With a contribution by
Andrew Symon RGN RM MA(Hons) PhD
Senior Lecturer, School of Nursing and Midwifery, The University of Dundee, Scotland, UK

Foreword by
Harry Gee MD MRCOG
Medical Director, Education and Resource Centre, The University of Birmingham, Birmingham Women's Healthcare NHS Trust

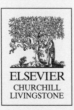

ELSEVIER
CHURCHILL
LIVINGSTONE

EDINBURGH LONDON NEW YORK OXFORD PHILADELPHIA ST LOUIS SYDNEY TORONTO 2005

ELSEVIER
CHURCHILL
LIVINGSTONE

First Edition 1992
Second Edition 1999
Third Edition 2005

ISBN 0 443 100667

British Library Cataloguing in Publication Data
A catalogue record for this book is available from the British Library

Library of Congress Cataloging in Publication Data
A catalog record for this book is available from the Library of Congress

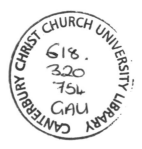
The
publisher's
policy is to use
**paper manufactured
from sustainable forests**

Printed in China

CONTENTS

It is in everyone's interest to detect and prevent the ill-effects of hypoxia on the fetus. Despite various approaches, heart rate monitoring remains the most convenient and well-tried method. In *CTG Made Easy* the authors provide an aid to more accurate interpretation of heart rate patterns.

CTG monitoring provides an indirect assessment of fetal well being. Heart rate control is complex involving neurological, endocrine and local mechanisms. The neurological control is mediated by interactions within the brainstem between afferent sensory systems (e.g. baroreceptors, chemoreceptors), higher centres (affected by behavioural states), centres controlling other vital systems (e.g. respiratory activity, thermoregulation) and the efferents via the parasympathetic and sympathetic autonomic nervous systems. It is not the purpose of this Foreword to describe the neurophysiology of heart rate control but only to illustrate its complexity and to demonstrate that the CTG is a relatively simple reflection of fetal condition. Our understanding of the physiological mechanisms has been gleaned from painstaking experimentation, usually testing one part of the system at a time. Even with precise understanding of the response of a single system it can be difficult to predict how the whole organism will respond when several interact with each other. Furthermore, the response of the fetus to hypoxia will depend upon its initial condition which, in turn, will

determine its ability to adapt or mount defence mechanisms. Thus, a growth-restricted fetus with little energy reserve is unlikely to withstand the ill-effects of hypoxia as readily as its well-nourished counterpart and be much more labile in its response.

As a general rule, a normal CTG gives sound re-assurance that the fetus is well at the time of recording. However, since physiological responses may produce abnormalities, an abnormal CTG may, or may not, represent compromise. Thus, the negative predictive value for pathology is good but the positive prediction, poor. This combination risks over-intervention and, even in the most skilled hands, the diagnosis of fetal compromise has to be resolved by further testing with, for example, fetal blood sampling. However, accurate interpretation of CTGs is the starting point and should be warmly welcomed to improve surveillance and avoid unnecessary intervention.

This edition has some important additions and the reorganisation of case studies makes *CTG Made Easy* even more relevant.

Birmingham, 2004
Harry Gee

For those not familiar with the origin of the book the idea of a case study approach to aid the interpretation of cardiotocographs arose in 1986 as a result of the 'Teaching and Assessing in Clinical Practice' course for midwives. A teaching package was produced containing a number of case histories including a section on the cardiotocograph followed by an analysis and description of the management instituted at the time. The package was used extensively in a number of delivery suites by midwives and doctors, initiating lively discussion. We know, from the comments of many doctors and midwives in the UK, that *CTG Made Easy* is used widely, arouses debate and aids learning. The book has an international readership and has been translated into German and Chinese.

In this the third edition we continue to follow the format followed previously but with a number of revisions and additions. In Part 1 we have included some of the issues surrounding the assessment of fetal well being in labour setting CTG within a wider perspective. Important documents and reports relevant to this are highlighted. Part 3, Litigation and Risk Management, with its use of legal case studies to illustrate important lessons has been updated. The Case studies section, Part 4, has been reviewed, some have been excluded and new ones inserted. Part 5 has been expanded and re-titled Good practice guide and contains some practical guidance, the risk assessment chart and some useful websites. We would welcome your comments on any aspect of the book particularly if you have any useful guides to good practice that could be included in future editions. We hope you find the changes helpful and that they will inform your judgements and decision making in practice.

Birmingham 2004
Christine Henderson
Susan Gauge

ACKNOWLEDGEMENTS

We would like to thank all those who have helped in the production of the book, especially midwives Annette Gough and Jennifer Henry, who were involved with the initial teaching package on which the book was based. We would also like to acknowledge the special contribution of the midwives and doctors on the delivery suite at the Birmingham Women's Healthcare NHS Trust, in particular Judith Weaver, Consultant Obstetrician, and Harold Gee, Clinical Director, for his support. Judith Weaver sadly died suddenly, just before this edition of the book was completed. We would like to dedicate this third edition to her in remembrance of all the support she has shown to many midwives and doctors over the years and the encouragement she has given to us in the development of this book.

INTRODUCTION

One of the questions uppermost in the minds of women, midwives and obstetricians during the course of labour tends to be 'is the baby alright?' One method of determining fetal well being during labour and delivery is monitoring of the fetal heart rate. The two main methods are intermittent and continuous, both can be achieved by using a variety of monitoring equipment. None of these are without their own risks and it is important to ensure that the most suitable method is offered to women dependant upon whether they are deemed to be at high or low risk of complications occurring during labour. In order to safeguard women, their babies and professionals, evidence-based guidelines should be in place to support practice and professionals must be confident and competent in the interpretation of the data produced, recognising the abnormal and initiating the correct management.

A number of texts are already in existence which describe in detail fetal physiology and monitoring techniques. It is not intended within this book to cover the same ground as these texts, but to complement them by initiating discussion relating to the interpretation of CTGs. It is hoped that this will be achieved by providing a series of examples of CTGs produced during labour.

The interpretation of antenatal CTGs differs from that of those produced during labour. In the absence of the stresses of labour, CTG abnormalities have a different significance and for this reason they have been excluded from this book.

This book is aimed at those with some knowledge and experience of fetal heart rate monitoring during labour and is divided into 5 parts.

Part 1 has been revised and includes information relating to intermittent auscultation and maintaining expertise, the reference list has also been updated to reflect current guidelines and reports.

Part 2 contains details of interpretation of CTGs with examples of a variety of fetal heart rate abnormalities.

Part 3, litigation and risk management highlights important aspects of fetal monitoring and presents some legal cases to illustrate the complexities of this practice. A reference list and extended bibliography are included at the end of this part.

Part 4 contains a series of case histories with a portion of the CTG. A set of questions to ask concerning the CTG are raised for consideration by the reader/group with the opportunity to make notes. An analysis and the management actually instigated at the time is stated. New CTGs have been added and they have been subdivided into sections. A new section, Miscellaneous, has been added for this edition.

A number of examples within this book show CTGs with data obtained by means of a fetal scalp electrode and in some cases contractions monitored by means of an intra uterine pressure catheter. We would acknowledge that in current practice these methods are infrequently, if ever, now used. However for the purpose of the interpretation of the CTG, the method by which they have been obtained in these instances is not important.

Part 5 has been expanded from the risk assessment chart to a guide to good practice. This section introduces a number of ways to develop good practice initiatives and gives examples of two such developments in current clinical practice. The risk assessment chart has been updated from the second edition and a list of useful web addresses is included.

The value of this book will be in the richness of discussions arising from the case studies as presented. Highlighting good practice may lead to further developments and review of existing guidelines. The benefits of this will only add to what every mother and baby deserves — practice that is safe, of the highest standard and results in an emotionally satisfying experience.

PART I

Assessing fetal well being

INTRODUCTION

Continuous monitoring of the fetal heart rate during labour became a widespread practice during the 1970s and has remained an accepted technique for assessing fetal well being in labour until relatively recently. Attitudes towards fetal monitoring have altered as more research findings are published and reviewed highlighting both the beneficial and detrimental effects of continuous electronic fetal heart rate monitoring (EFM) (RCOG 2001a, Vintzileos et al 1995, Neilson & Grant 1993).

One of the main debates in this arena is the method of EFM used in labour for women categorised as low risk or non complex. It has been shown that for these mothers continuous EFM confers no benefit to the fetus (MacDonald et al 1985) and increases operative interventions (NICE 2004, Mongelli et al 1997, Supplee & Vezeau 1996, Thacker et al 1995).

The National Sentinel Caesarean Section Audit Report (RCOG 2001b) identified that the most frequently cited primary reason for performing a caesarean section was presumed fetal compromise. There is evidence to suggest that maternal morbidity and mortality can be adversely affected by caesarean section (NICE 2004) and, while maternal mortality rates continue to fall, there is an indirect link between death rates and caesarean section (Hall 2001). Any unnecessary procedure that may increase the risk of caesarean section, such as continuous EFM in a low risk woman, would therefore best be avoided.

Grant (1989), stated that the use of electronic fetal monitoring, with present knowledge, should be restricted to high risk or complex cases. Indeed the most recent guidelines developed by the Royal College of Obstetricians and Gynaecologists (RCOG 2001a) and inherited by The National Institute for Clinical Excellence (NICE 2001) reiterate the findings of these earlier studies.

It is important that women have adequate information and are involved in the decision making process about the method of fetal monitoring used during labour (NHS Litigation Authority 2004, NICE 2001, DoH 1993). An Audit Commission report in 1997 highlighted that less than 20% of women felt that they had been involved in decisions about fetal monitoring (Audit Commission 1997). Professionals involved in caring for women in labour must be aware of the most recent recommendations and evidence relating to fetal monitoring in order for valid consent to be obtained.

The Department of Health have produced a guide to consent for treatment which reiterates this and other factors which must be taken into account (DoH 2001a). Midwives in particular are urged to be as up to date as possible with current evidence in order to promote physiological childbirth (DoH 2003). To assist midwives with this task MIDIRS produce a range of informed-choice information for women and professionals, including one relating to fetal heart rate monitoring in labour (MIDIRS 2003). The importance of promoting evidence-based practice is also laid down in the Midwives Rules and Standards (NMC 2004) and Code of Professional Conduct (NMC 2002), with Supervisors of Midwives holding responsibility for supporting midwives in their delivery of the service. (West Midlands LSA Consortium 2003).

Concerns have been expressed regarding the routine use of continuous EFM during labour (Cooke 1992, Evans 1992). Dover and Gauge (1995) found that, when questioned, midwives stated that intermittent auscultation was their preferred method of fetal monitoring for low risk women in labour; however, when reviewing clinical practice it appeared that continuous monitoring by means of abdominal transducers was more widely used than was suggested. Another study, relating to practice and attitudes, highlights the ambiguity of the professionals' definition of intermittent fetal monitoring (Birch & Thompson 1997).

The Royal College of Midwives (RCM) Standing Practice Group (1994) advised midwives to analyse their reasons for using continuous EFM on women in normal labour and to assess procedures in their workplaces. Munro et al (2002) reported positive progress at two maternity units who demonstrated an increase in the rate of intermittent auscultation for low risk women in labour. They also noted that midwives' attitudes towards methods of fetal heart rate monitoring were changing, whilst acknowledging that change in practice does take a considerable time. Costello and Munro (2003) reported from an audit of the NICE guidelines for fetal monitoring in practice that although there are some areas that require further work, it was encouraging to note that intermittent auscultation was used by the majority of midwives.

For the first time in many years we are seeing a move towards non intervention for low risk women in relation to fetal monitoring in labour. Midwives are being encouraged by national guidelines to use their traditional skills to be with women in labour and childbirth. However, there remains a duty of care for the women who fall into high risk or complex categories. In light of available evidence it is still recommended that fetal well being in labour should be assessed by continuous EFM (NICE 2001). The optimum outcome for mother and baby relies heavily upon the interpretation of the resulting data in the form of the cardiotocograph (CTG).

While the primary aim of this book remains to encourage standardised interpretation of the CTG, a small section on intermittent auscultation (IA), to the low risk woman, has been included.

INTERMITTENT AUSCULTATION

For low risk women, intermittent auscultation for the assessment of fetal well being in labour should be offered and recommended by the professional involved in her care (NICE 2001). This may be by means of the Pinard stethoscope or a hand held Doppler. The latter may have the benefit of being more comfortable for the woman in allowing her to remain in her chosen position for labour, while still allowing the midwife access to estimate the fetal heart rate reliably (Mainstone 2004, Mahomed et al 1994, Garcia et al 1985).

Murphy-Black (1991) observed that midwives appeared to be losing their traditional skills in auscultation of the fetal heart with a Pinard stethoscope. Wickham (2002a, 2002b) has tried to redress this by publishing tips for midwives in the use of the Pinard stethoscope. She also reports that midwives are aware of the potential increased risk of caesarean section when using Doppler (Wickham 2002b); a finding reported by Mohamed et al (1994). Harrison (2004) discusses the instruments used for auscultation, concluding that the hand held Doppler has advantages over the Pinard stethoscope, however later correspondence gives a differing point of view (Soltani & Shallow 2004).

There is also some debate regarding how the fetal heart rate is counted during auscultation. Current practice recommends counting the heart rate for a full minute, while it has been reported that a multi count method may be more accurate in identifying periodic changes (Schifrin 1992, Paine et al 1986). Concerns have been expressed about the ability to detect variability by auscultation (Harrison 2004), although some midwives feel confident in their abilities to detect variations from normal, both baseline and periodic changes, when using a Pinard stethoscope (Association of Radical Midwives 2000).

Current practice recommendations for intermittent auscultation as a means of assessing fetal well being in labour have been issued by NICE and are as follows:

> In the active stages of labour, intermittent auscultation should occur after a contraction, for a minimum of 60 seconds, and at least:
>
> Every 15 minutes in the first stage
> Every 5 minutes in the second stage.
> (NICE 2001)

These guidelines do not specify an instrument of choice, which ever is most convenient and acceptable to the woman and midwife would appear appropriate. This does provide midwives with an ideal opportunity to develop and maintain their skills in auscultation with a Pinard stethoscope as, in the absence of technology and batteries, it is the only tool available. More importantly it will encourage the passing down of the skills to students, the midwives and obstetricians of the future.

There a number of points to consider when using intermittent auscultation:

- It is important that women are correctly identified as falling into a low risk category for labour.
- Risk factors can change at any point during labour necessitating a move to continuous EFM.
- Maternal pulse should be assessed and recorded prior to auscultation. If there is any doubt about the rate being heard they should be assessed simultaneously.
- Any concerns regarding the fetal heart rate should be documented and EFM commenced. A return to intermittent auscultation can be instigated providing normal parameters have been met on the CTG.
- There will be no print out, accurate documentation is essential. This can prove to be difficult, particularly in the second stage of labour (see Good Practice Guide).

While there are still some issues relating to intermittent auscultation that would benefit from further research, it is recognised as a safe method of assessing fetal well being in labour for low risk women (NICE 2001). There is evidence to suggest that practice changes are being adopted, although it is recognised that this takes time. While it is excellent that we are no longer totally reliant upon machines, it has to be remembered that the technology still has its place in clinical care. The important factor is having sufficient knowledge and experience to use it when required and confidence in intermittent auscultation where indicated.

THE CARDIOTOCOGRAPH (CTG)

Given the fact that continuous EFM is still used as a method of assessing the well being of the fetus during labour, it is imperative that midwives and medical staff feel confident in correctly interpreting the data on the CTG and instigating the correct management when fetal heart rate abnormalities are detected. Reports from a confidential enquiry concentrating on intrapartum deaths highlights suboptimal intrapartum care in 75.6% of cases, the most common criticism being the failure to recognise abnormalities occurring on the CTG (CESDI 1997). Another previous study concerned with obstetric litigation also highlighted failure to respond to CTG abnormalities as a problem (Ennis & Vincent 1990). The variability in interpretation between observers is a well-recognised problem when analysing data on the CTG (Blix et al 2003). Developments continue in order to improve the analysis of fetal heart rate patterns and subsequent support for clinical decisions (Greene 1996), and have been widely discussed (Richens 2001, Jibodu & Arulkumaran 2000).

Having stated that correct interpretation of the data on the CTG is vital to assisting decisions regarding management of labour, it is important that this information is not used in isolation. The progress being made in labour, the amount and colour of any liquor draining and the use of Syntocinon (oxytocin) to augment uterine contractions must be taken into account. Failure to observe all of these factors has been noted to be a common problem (Gibb 1997). The Royal College of Obstetricians and Gynaecologists (RCOG 1993) recommend that fetal heart rate monitoring should only be used when facilities are available for fetal blood pH measurements, and, ideally, estimation of PO_2, PCO_2 and base excess, to allow confirmation of suspected fetal compromise as shown by the CTG.

It has been established that the predictive value of continuous EFM is improved by the use of fetal blood sampling and analysis during labour (NICE 2001). However, this procedure requires skill and can often be uncomfortable for the woman and has the potential for both false positive and negative results (Balen 1993). Despite this, NICE (2001) recommend that whenever EFM is in use there must be ready access to fetal blood sampling facilities. Westgate et al (1994) have also demonstrated that umbilical cord blood acid–base balance at the time of delivery, although not a predictor, can assist with the identification of those babies that may be at risk of neonatal morbidity. NICE (2001) list the situations when cord blood analysis should be performed.

Interpretation

The interpretation of antenatal and labour CTGs differ. Certain fetal heart rate abnormalities, mainly decelerations, cannot be classified in the absence of uterine contractions, and indeed the physiological explanation for their occurrence may be different. Also during labour the maternal and fetal energy and oxygen requirements change, which places the fetus in a stressful situation. The fetus, in normal circumstances, is able to cope with these changes; however, if a fetus is already compromised before labour begins, the additional stress of uterine contractions diminishes the energy and oxygen flow from the mother to such an extent that fetal compromise can occur. The following must be considered:

1. Pre-existence of any medical conditions in the mother, e.g.
   Diabetes mellitus
   Renal disease
2. Existence of any pregnancy-related diseases, e.g.
   Pregnancy-induced hypertension
   Rhesus incompatibility
3. Identified risk factors occurring in pregnancy, e.g.
   Intrauterine growth retardation
   Fetal abnormality
   Antepartum haemorrhage
4. Gestational period
5. Progress in labour
6. Any drugs administered to the mother, e.g.
   Benzodiazapines (temazepam)
   Tocolytic agents (salbutamol, terbutaline)
   Analgesics (pethidine, diamorphine)
   Anaesthesia (epidural or spinal block)

Self administered drugs (nicotine, alcohol, cannabis, heroin, etc.)
7. Posture of the mother throughout the CTG — lying supine will cause a decrease in uterine blood flow, and hence a decrease in oxygen and energy transfer to the fetus.

It is necessary to record certain information on the CTG, to aid in both identification and interpretation:

1. Name and registration number of the mother.
2. Date and time of any recording. If the monitor prints this out automatically it must be checked for accuracy, particularly around times of clock changes to and from British Summer Time.
3. The maternal pulse rate at the beginning of the CTG.
4. Posture of the mother and changes that occur.
5. Speed of the paper, i.e. either 1 cm/min or 3 cm/min.
6. All drugs administered to the mother.
7. Vaginal examinations and findings, e.g. cervical dilation, artificial rupture of membranes, state of any liquor observed.
8. Blood pressure recordings before and after epidural analgesia.
9. Method of monitoring the fetal heart, i.e. internal by means of a fetal scalp electrode, or external by means of an abdominal transducer.

In order to analyse a CTG accurately, the recording must be of good quality. A poor-quality CTG is impossible to interpret; fetal heart rate abnormalities can be missed or mistakenly identified. Uterine activity must be monitored adequately in conjunction with the fetal heart rate. Fetal heart rate abnormalities that occur are classified by relating them to the uterine contractions. If they are not recorded, then an accurate analysis becomes impossible.

It is advisable to establish the presence of the fetal heart with a Pinard stethoscope prior to commencing a CTG (Medical Devices Agency 2002). If there is any doubt as to the rate of the fetal heart recording on the CTG, it is advisable to auscultate with a Pinard stethoscope or hand held Doppler and write the rate on the CTG. It is also important to document the maternal pulse prior to any EFM recording and at regular intervals during labour, as there have been instances where stillbirths have occurred in the presence of CTGs interpreted as normal (Medical Devices Agency 2002). NICE (2001) recommend that the maternal pulse is palpated simultaneously to auscultation of the fetal heart to ensure that they are different.

It is possible for the fetal heart rate monitor to either double count a low fetal heart rate, or to half count a high rate, e.g. a true rate of 60 beats per minute (b.p.m.) may record as 120 b.p.m. or a true rate of 180 b.p.m. may record as 90 b.p.m.

Although unusual, it is possible for the monitor to count the maternal pulse rate. This may occur after the application of a fetal scalp electrode if the fetus is dead (Herbert et al 1987), or with an abdominal transducer even if the fetus is alive.

MAINTAINING EXPERTISE

The CTG only becomes a valuable method of monitoring and assessing fetal well being in labour if the professionals involved are able to interpret the data correctly and have an understanding of the underlying normal physiology and that of abnormalities that can occur. This requires regular training and updating in the interpretation of CTGs. Recommendations of updating at intervals between 6 months and yearly have been made (CESDI 1997, RCOG 1993) and reiterated in subsequent documents (NHS Litigation Authority 2004, NICE 2001, CESDI 2000).

Clinical risk management is becoming inherent within midwifery and obstetric practice (Wilson & Symon 2002). Certainly incorrect interpretation of CTGs and ensuing actions place women and babies at a potentially high risk of harm. It is the responsibility of each practitioner to ensure that they remain clinically updated (NMC 2004) and co-operate with Department of Health guidance relating to minimising risk for women and babies (DoH 2000, 2001b).

Each individual will have a preferred method of learning and suggestions for updating include:

- Attendance at study days with a particular theme of CTG interpretation.
- Regular multidisciplinary meetings to discuss CTG interpretation.
- Use of interactive computer software such as that described by Beckley et al (2000).
- Involvement in setting guidelines for fetal monitoring.

A record of attendance at all training and updating of CTG interpretation should be maintained and help sought by professionals who have difficulty accessing such training. Training and updating in the use of intermittent auscultation is also important to ensure that correct techniques are used and that guidelines are being followed. It is also recommended that training sessions include information on documentation and storage relating to CTGs (NICE 2001, CESDI 2000).

The main message here is really that in order to maintain a high standard of care it is imperative that professionals remain up to date with current recommendations regarding methods of fetal monitoring and the interpretation of the resulting data. Every individual has the responsibility to ensure that they have this knowledge and are able to use it in their clinical practice.

REFERENCES

Association of Radical Midwives (2000) Hearing variability. Midwifery Matters (84) Spring

Audit Commission (1997) First class delivery. Improving maternity services in England and Wales. Audit Commission, London

Balen A (1993) The value of cardiotocography for intrapartum monitoring. British Journal of Midwifery 1(4): 174–176

Beckley S, Stenhouse E, Greene K (2000) The development and evaluation of a computer-assisted teaching programme for intrapartum fetal monitoring. British Journal of Obstetrics and Gynaecology 107(11): 1138–1144

Birch L, Thompson B (1997) Survey into fetal monitoring practices and attitudes. British Journal of Midwifery 5(12): 732–736

Blix E, Sviggum O, Sofie Kass K, Oian P (2003) Inter-observer variation in assessment of 845 labour admission tests: comparison between midwives and obstetricians in the clinical setting and two experts. British Journal of Obstetrics and Gynaecology 110(1): 1–5

CESDI (Confidential Enquiry into Stillbirths and Deaths in Infancy) (1997) Fourth Annual Report. Maternal and Child Health Research Consortium, London

CESDI (Confidential Enquiry into Stillbirths and Deaths in Infancy) (2000) Seventh Annual Report. Maternal and Child Health Research Consortium, London

Cooke P (1992) Fetal monitoring – a questionable practice? Modern Midwife 2(2): 8–11

Costello J, Munro J (2003) An audit of NICE guidelines for the use of electronic fetal monitoring in labour. MIDIRS Midwifery Digest 13(1): 66–68

DoH (Department of Health) (1993) Changing childbirth. Report of the Expert Maternity Group. HMSO, London

DoH (Department of Health) (2000) An organisation with a memory. DoH, London

DoH (Department of Health) (2001a) Reference guide to consent for examination and treatment. DoH, London

DoH (Department of Health) (2001b) Building a safer NHS for patients. DoH, London

DoH (Department of Health) (2003) Delivering the best. Midwives contribution to the NHS Plan. DoH, London

Dover S L, Gauge S M (1995) Fetal monitoring –midwives' attitudes. Midwifery 11(1): 18–27

Ennis M, Vincent C A (1990) Obstetric accidents: a review of 64 cases. British Medical Journal 300: 1365–1367

Evans S (1992) The value of cardiotocograph monitoring in midwifery. Midwives Chronicle 105(1248): 4–10

Garcia J, Corry M, MacDonald D, Elbourne D, Grant A (1985) Mothers' views on continuous electronic fetal heart rate monitoring and intermittent auscultation in a randomised controlled trial. Birth 21(2): 79–85

Gibb D (1997) Really understanding the cardiotocograph (CTG). Professional Care of Mother and Child 7(5): 125–128

Grant A (1989) Monitoring the fetus during labour. In: Chalmers I, Enkin M, Keirse M (eds) Effective care in pregnancy and childbirth. Oxford University Press, Oxford, p 846–888

Grant J M (1991) The fetal heart trace is normal, isn't it? Lancet 337: 215–218

Greene K R (1996) Intelligent fetal heart rate computer systems in intrapartum surveillance. Current Opinion in Obstetrics and Gynaecology 8(2): 123–127

Hall M H (2001) Caesarean section. In: Why mothers die 1997 – 1999. The confidential enquiries into maternal deaths in the United Kingdom. RCOG Press, London, p 317–325

Harrison J (2004) Auscultation: the art of listening. Midwives 7(2):64–69

Herbert W N P, Stuart N N, Butler L S (1987) Electronic fetal heart rate monitoring with intrauterine demise. Journal of Obstetric, Gynecologic and Neonatal Nursing 16(4): 249–252

Jibodu OA, Arulkumaran S (2000) Intrapartum fetal surveillance. Current Opinion in Obstetrics and Gynaecology 12(2): 123–127

MacDonald D, Grant A, Sheridan-Pereira M, Boylen P, Chalmers I (1985) The Dublin randomised controlled trial of intrapartum fetal heart rate monitoring. American Journal of Obstetrics and Gynecology 52: 524–539

Mahomed K, Nyoni R, Mulambo T, Kausle J, Jacobus E (1994) Randomised controlled trial of intrapartum fetal heart rate monitoring. British Medical Journal 308(6927): 497–500

Mainston A (2004) The use of doppler in fetal monitoring. British Journal of Midwifery 12(2): 78–83

Medical Devices Agency (2002) Cardiotocograph (CTG) monitoring of fetus during labour-update. Safety Notice MDS SN2002(23) August 2002. MDA, London

MIDIRS (2003) Fetal heart rate monitoring in labour. Informed choice for professionals. MIDIRS, Bristol

Mongelli M, Chung T K H, Chang A M Z (1997) Obstetric intervention and benefit in conditions of very low prevalence. British Journal of Obstetrics and Gynaecology 104(7): 771–774

Munro J, Ford H, Scott A, Furnival E, Andrews S, Grayson A (2002) Action research project responding to midwives views of different methods of fetal monitoring in labour. MIDIRS Midwifery Digest 12(4): 495–498

Murphy-Black T (1991) Fetal monitoring in labour. Nursing Times 87(28): 58–59

Neilson J P, Grant A M (1993) The randomised trials of intrapartum electronic fetal heart rate monitoring. In: Spencer J A D, Ward R H T (eds) Intrapartum fetal surveillance. RCOG Press, London, p 77–93

NHS Litigation Authority (2004) Clinical negligence scheme for Trusts. Clinical risk management standards for the maternity services. NHS Litigation Authority, London

NICE (2001) The use of electronic fetal monitoring. Inherited clinical guideline C. NICE, London

NICE (2004) Caesarean section, clinical guideline. NICE, London

NMC (2002) Code of professional conduct. NMC, London

NMC (2004) Midwives rules and standards. NMC, London

Paine L L, Johnson T R B , Turner M H, Payton R G (1986) Auscultated fetal heart rate accelerations: part two: an alternative to the non stress test. Journal of Nurse-Midwifery. 31(2): 73 – 77

RCM Standing Practice Group (1994) Paper 1: To monitor or not to monitor: the midwife's use of electrocardiographic forms of monitoring the fetus in labour. Midwives Chronicle 107(1276): 189

RCOG (Royal College of Obstetricians and Gynaecologists) (1993) Twenty sixth RCOG Study Group. Intrapartum fetal surveillance. RCOG Press, London

RCOG (Royal College of Obstetricians and Gynaecologists) (2001a) The use of electronic fetal monitoring. Evidence based guideline no 8. RCOG Press, London

RCOG (Royal College of Obstetricians and Gynaecologists) (2001b) The National Sentinel Caesarean Section Audit Report. RCOG Press, London

Richens Y (2001) New horizons on intrapartum electronic fetal monitoring. British Journal of Midwifery 9(9): 584–585

Schifrin B S, Amsel J, Burdof G (1992) The accuracy of auscultatory detection of fetal cardiac decelerations: a computer simulation. American Journal of Obstetrics and Gynaecology. 166(2): 566 – 576

Soltani H, Shallow H (2004) Re :auscultation. Letters Midwives 7(4): 172

Supplee R B, Vezeau T M (1996) Continuous electronic fetal monitoring: does it belong in low-risk births? American Journal of Maternal/Child Nursing 21(6): 301–306

Thacker S B, Stroup D F, Peterson H B (1995) Efficacy and safety of intrapartum electronic fetal monitoring: an update. Obstetrics and Gynaecology 86(4): 613–620

Vintzileos A M, Nochimson D J, Guzman E R, Knuppel R A, Lake M, Schifrin B S (1995) Intrapartum electronic fetal heart rate monitoring versus intermittent auscultation: a meta-analysis. Obstetrics and Gynaecology 85(1): 149–154

West Midlands Local Supervising Authority Consortium (2003) Standards and guidelines for supervisors of midwives. West Midlands LSA, Worcester

Westgate J, Garibaldi J, Greene K (1994) Umbilical cord blood gas analysis at delivery: a time for quality data. British Journal of Obstetrics and Gynaecology 101: 1054–1063

Wickham S (2002a) Pinard wisdom. The Practising Midwife 5(9): 21

Wickham S (2002b) Pinard wisdom part 2. The Practising Midwife 5(10): 35

Wilson J H, Symon A (2002) Clinical risk management in midwifery. Books for Midwives, Oxford

PART 2

Interpretation of the CTG

When interpreting a CTG, there are four main points to consider relating to the fetal heart rate:

Basic patterns
1. Baseline heart rate
2. Variability.

Periodic changes
3. Accelerations
4. Decelerations.

In normal circumstances:

1. The baseline fetal heart rate is 110–160 b.p.m.
2. The variability is 5–15 b.p.m.
3. Accelerations may or may not occur in response to uterine contractions or fetal movements
4. No decelerations occur.

Figure 2.1 shows an example of a normal CTG.

BASIC PATTERNS

Baseline fetal heart rate

This illustrates the rate of the fetal heart, which is controlled mainly by the autonomic nervous system. Sympathetic activity results in tachycardia, while parasympathetic activity, mainly the vagus nerve, results in bradycardia. In normal circumstances, the vagal activity is dominant, exerting a constant slowing of the heart rate, stabilising it at 110–160 b.p.m. The baseline fetal heart is also controlled by receptors in the aortic arch:

1. Chemoreceptors, which are stimulated by changes in oxygen levels. An acute fall in oxygen levels leads to an increase in parasympathetic activity, resulting in a slowing of the heart rate. A more prolonged fall will lead to chronic changes and an increase in sympathetic activity, resulting in a rise in the heart rate.
2. Baroreceptors, which are stimulated by changes in arterial pressure. Hypertension leads to an increase in parasympathetic activity, resulting in a slowing of the heart rate. Hypotension leads to an increase in sympathetic activity, resulting in a rise in the heart rate.

The baseline heart rate is also related to gestational age and the maturity of the vagus nerve. The more mature the fetus, the more evident the slowing effect that the vagus nerve exerts upon the heart rate becomes.

Baseline bradycardia

Definition
Baseline bradycardia is defined as being a persistently low baseline of below 110 b.p.m.

Causes
Many baseline bradycardias have no identifiable cause but there are certain factors that need to be taken into consideration:

1. *Gestational age of greater than 40 weeks.* Some postmature fetuses have a marked vagal tone, causing a slowing of the heart rate, and can show a baseline bradycardia of 90–110 b.p.m.
2. *Cord compression.* In cases of acute hypoxia and cord compression a change in the baseline is usually evident from within a normal range to bradycardia.
3. *Congenital heart malformations.*
4. *Certain drugs*, e.g. benzodiazepines.

Management
If fetal hypoxia is suspected, a fetal blood sample should be obtained to estimate the pH value and base deficit of the fetal blood. Vaginal examination should be performed to exclude umbilical cord prolapse. Providing that there are no further fetal heart rate abnormalities occurring on the CTG, careful observation is all that is necessary.

Baseline tachycardia

Definition
Baseline tachycardia is defined as being a persistently high baseline of above 160 b.p.m.

Causes
1. *Excessive fetal movements or fetal stimulation.* If the fetus is very active during the period that the CTG is being performed, the fetal heart may not be showing a true baseline. This should be

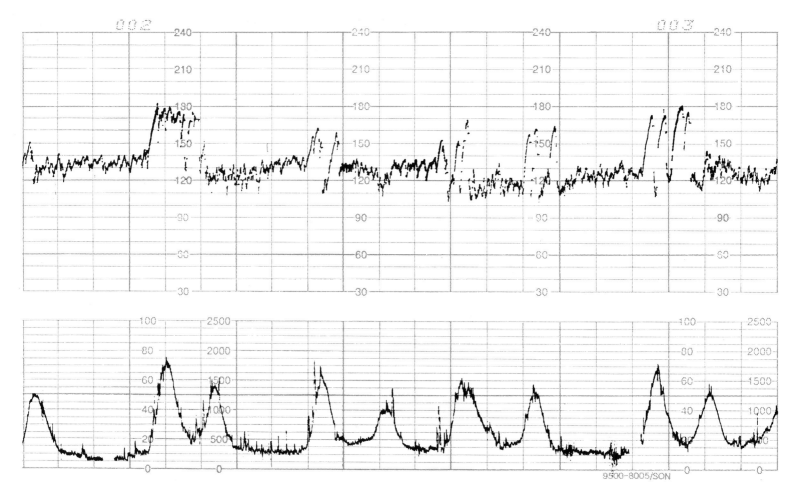

Fig. 2.1 *Normal CTG. Fetal heart recorded using fetal scalp electrode. Contractions recorded using an external transducer. Baseline 125–135 b.p.m.; baseline variability 5–15 b.p.m.; no decelerations, accelerations with some contractions.*

classed as reactivity, but can be mistakenly diagnosed as fetal tachycardia.

2. *Maternal stress and anxiety.* If the mother is in a stressful situation, or has a high anxiety level, she will release catecholamines, thereby stimulating the sympathetic nervous system, resulting in an increase in both maternal and fetal heart rates.

3. *Gestational age.* A fetus at a gestational age of 32 weeks or below can show a baseline tachycardia due to the immaturity of the vagus nerve. The sympathetic nervous system is dominant, resulting in a persistently high fetal heart rate.

4. *Maternal pyrexia.* This is usually associated with maternal tachycardia. Mothers can develop a pyrexia in labour unrelated to infection, particularly if epidural analgesia is used, or if the labour has been long, and signs of maternal distress or obstructed labour are evident. However, with modern management of labour, this should rarely, if ever, be seen. When fetal tachycardia is diagnosed, infection should always be considered.

5. *Fetal infection.* During infection, oxygen requirements are raised. The heart rate rises to increase the oxygen transfer around the body.

6. *Chronic hypoxia.* Chronic changes in the levels of oxygen tension lead to an increase in the sympathetic activity, resulting in a rise in the heart rate. In this instance, the tachycardia may also be complicated by a decrease in variability.

7. *Fetal hormones.* The fetus, in response to stressful situations, e.g. a decrease in oxygen levels, can produce hormones from the adrenal glands, adrenaline and noradrenaline. Their effect is similar to an increase in sympathetic activity, that is, a rise in the heart rate. Therefore, a baseline tachycardia can also be the initial response to fetal hypoxia.

Management

1. Record maternal temperature and pulse rate to exclude pyrexia. If infection is suspected then appropriate treatment should be initiated.

2. If fetal hypoxia is suspected, a fetal blood sample should be obtained to assess the pH value and base excess of the fetal blood, particularly if any other fetal heart rate abnormalities are present. The value of fetal blood sampling in the presence of maternal pyrexia is questionable.

Providing that no further fetal heart rate abnormalities are present, careful observation of the trace is all that is necessary.

Variability

Definition

Variability is due to interaction between all the systems previously described and occurs as a result of the beat-to-beat changes in the heart rate. Normal variability is between 5–15 b.p.m. (see Fig. 2.1).

Variability can be measured by analysing a 1-minute portion of a CTG, and assessing the amplitude of change in the heart rate during that period, i.e. the difference in the number of beats per minute of the fetal heart from the highest rate to the lowest rate (any accelerations and decelerations should be excluded; e.g. if the highest rate is 160 b.p.m. and the lowest rate is 155 b.p.m. the difference. is 5 b.p.m.).

Aetiology

Variability represents the constant interaction of the sympathetic and parasympathetic nervous systems as they determine the appropriate heart rate and cardiac output in response to constant minor changes in venous return and metabolic demands of the fetus. Normal variability represents an intact nervous pathway through the cerebral cortex, midbrain, vagus nerve and cardiac conduction system. Variability is likely to occur as a result of numerous inputs transmitted through these areas of the nervous system.

Variability can be analysed as being:

1. Normal
2. Increased
3. Decreased.

In order for beat to beat variability to be interpreted correctly, the heart rate must be

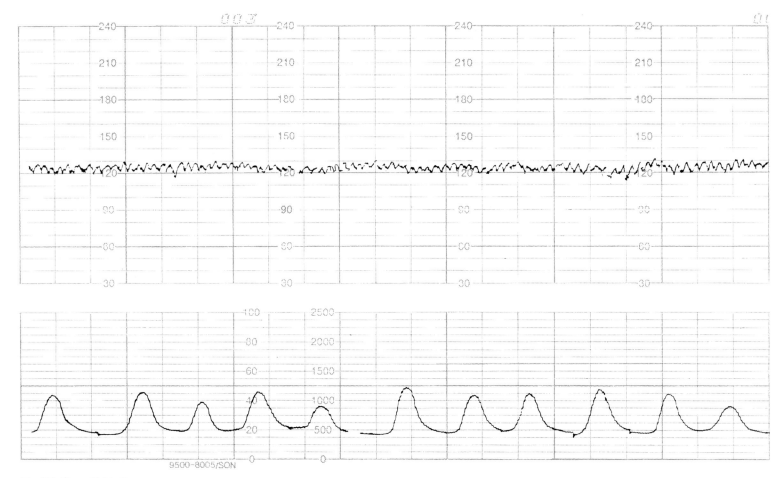

Fig. 2.2 *Sinusoidal pattern.*

monitored on a beat-to-beat basis, by the use of direct fetal electrocardiograph monitoring, achieved by the application of a fetal scalp electrode. When monitoring the fetal heart by means of an abdominal transducer, the monitor recognises each heart beat from a series of echoes and uses the strongest of these to measure the heart rate. The strongest echo may not occur at the same time in every heart beat, resulting in inaccurate measurements of the beat to beat fetal heart rate variability. Measurement of variability in this instance should be expressed as 10 beats and not 10 beats per minute.

Increased variability

Causes
The initial fetal response to acute hypoxia may cause a transient increase in variability due to stimulation of the parasympathetic nervous system.

Decreased variability

Causes
1. *Fetal sleep*. During fetal sleep the CTG may give an appearance of decreased variability; this should not be confused with lack of reactivity. This pattern should not persist for longer than 40 minutes, after which time the variability should return to within normal limits.
2. *Administration of drugs to the mother*. Decreased variability can be seen following the administration of pethidine to the mother in labour, or of sedative drugs. This pattern should not persist for longer than 30–40 minutes. Variability should then return to normal.
3. *Gestational age*. The CTG of a fetus at a gestational age of less than 28–30 weeks may show decreased variability, most probably due to the immaturity of the autonomic nervous system.
4. *Severe hypoxia*. When the fetus is suffering from severe or chronic hypoxia the autonomic nervous system fails to respond to stress and the changes in venous return and metabolic demands of the fetus. This is due to a reduction in the transmission of impulses through the nervous system. In the presence of cerebral hypoxia, variability is often severely diminished or absent.

Management
When diminished variability is diagnosed on a CTG, providing any obvious causes, such as administration of pethidine, can be eliminated, fetal hypoxia must always be considered as a cause. Fetal blood sampling should be performed to assess the pH value and base excess of the blood.

The baseline fetal heart rate and variability together are useful indicators of fetal oxygenation. Normal variability represents a fully functioning nervous system. Even in the presence of other fetal heart rate abnormalities suggestive of hypoxia, if the variability is within normal limits, the outcome is usually good.

In the instance of chronic fetal cerebral hypoxia, a decrease or absence of variability may be the only fetal heart rate abnormality present.

Sinusoidal pattern
Sinusoidal patterns may not be viewed as a precise group by some, rather as a subgroup, as there is an increasing tendency today to analyse fetal heart rate according to the frequency of oscillations.

In a study by Young et al (1980) true sinusoidal patterns were uncommon, occurring in only 0.3% of monitored labours. Nonetheless, they do occur and it is important to recognise such a pattern when it occurs.

Definition
This pattern is identifiable by its distinctive smooth, undulating sine-wave-like baseline. Beat-to-beat variability is absent. Figure 2.2 shows an example CTG exhibiting a sinusoidal pattern.

Aetiology
It is thought that this pattern may be a result of cord compression, resulting in alternating hypervolaemia and hypovolaemia, or of a raised intraperitoneal pressure due to the presence of ascites, resulting in a reduction and

eventual cessation of umbilical venous blood flow. In both instances, significant fetal hypoxia will result (O'Connor et al 1980).

Causes
These would fall into three areas: severe hypoxia, anaemia and idiopathic.

Idiopathic. This pattern can be seen as a result of fetal thumb-sucking, and is sometimes seen following the administration of narcotic analgesia to the mother (Egley et al 1991). In these cases the pattern should not persist for longer than 20–30 minutes before a return to normal variability.

Anaemia. The fetus presenting as anaemic, particularly as a result of rhesus incompatibility, twin-to-twin transfusion or large fetomaternal bleed, may produce a sinusoidal pattern.

O'Connor et al (1980) point out, following a review of the literature, that sinusoidal tracings where the oscillations have an amplitude of 20 beats or more, and a frequency of 1–2 oscillations per minute are more suggestive of fetal hypoxia and are an indication for immediate delivery.

Sinusoidal traces where the amplitude of the oscillations is 10 beats or less, with a frequency of 3–5 per minute, may be due to fetal anaemia or thumb-sucking. They can be referred to as pseudosinusoidal and do not usually require immediate action. However, if other fetal heart rate abnormalities are present, delivery should not be delayed.

Management
This pattern should always be regarded as sinister until proven otherwise. A fetal blood sample should be obtained to assess the pH value and base excess of the fetal blood.

If the pattern persists it is an indication for immediate delivery.

PERIODIC CHANGES

Accelerations

Definition
An acceleration is an increase in the fetal heart rate of 15 b.p.m. or more, lasting for at least 15 seconds. Accelerations usually occur in a response to either a fetal movement or a uterine contraction. When accelerations occur the CTG is said to be reactive.

Aetiology
The reaction is caused by the interaction of the sympathetic and parasympathetic nervous systems as a result of an increase in metabolic demands of the fetus during an active phase, or during a uterine contraction in response to compression of the umbilical cord and fetal trunk.

Increased reactivity
This can be due to a period of excessive fetal movements. On analysis of the CTG, increased reactivity can be mistakenly identified as baseline tachycardia.

Decreased reactivity
This can be due to either a period of fetal sleep or the administration of sedation or analgesia to the mother. Methods of fetal stimulation, such as abdominal palpation or giving the mother cold water to drink, can evoke a response in the fetus.

It is important not to confuse decreased reactivity with decreased variability. A CTG can be non-reactive but still show variability within normal limits.

Decelerations
Decelerations of the fetal heart rate from the baseline can be classified into four types:

1. Early deceleration
2. Late deceleration
3. Variable deceleration
4. Prolonged deceleration.

The definition and physiological explanation for each type of deceleration is different. It is important to classify them accurately in order for the most effective management to be initiated. Uterine contractions must be monitored adequately in order for the deceleration to be classified.

Early decelerations
Definition. Early decelerations tend to be uniform in shape and occur with each contraction. They

often appear in a mirror image of the contraction. The onset of the deceleration is at the onset of the contraction. The heart rate reaches its lowest point at the peak of the contraction and has recovered to the baseline by the end of the contraction. The amplitude of the deceleration is 40 b.p.m. or less. Early decelerations are not commonly seen and care should be taken when diagnosing them on a CTG.

Figure 2.3 shows an example CTG exhibiting early decelerations.

Aetiology. Early decelerations are caused by compression of the fetal head during a contraction. Compression of the fetal head causes an increase in intracranial pressure and therefore a decrease in cerebral blood flow and oxygenation. The decrease in oxygen tension is detected by cerebral chemoreceptors, and parasympathetic activity is increased, resulting in a fall in the fetal heart rate. During head compression, pressure on the vagal centre in the brain may also occur, increasing parasympathetic activity.

These decelerations are caused by a mild, transient hypoxia and are not associated with a poor fetal outcome.

Management. This is aimed at relieving the pressure on the fetal head during a uterine contraction. Changing the maternal posture is normally all that is required.

Late decelerations

Definition. Late decelerations are usually uniform in shape, depth and occur after each contraction. Any deceleration whose lowest point occurs more than 15 seconds after the peak of the contraction is said to be late (for an example CTG, see Fig. 2.4).

Aetiology. Late decelerations arise as a result of a decrease in uterine blood flow and therefore oxygen transfer during a uterine contraction. The low oxygen tension is detected by chemoreceptors in the aortic arch, resulting in stimulation of the parasympathetic pathways and an increase in vagal activity, leading to a fall in the heart rate. The decelerations occur after the contraction owing to the time it takes for the circulating blood to reach the aortic arch from the placenta. In between the contractions the rate of oxygen transfer between the placenta and the fetus is adequate, and the fetal heart rate baseline and variability are normal, indicating adequate cerebral oxygenation. If, however, the fetus is already compromised, then the reduced amount of oxygen transferred during a contraction may not be sufficient to maintain myocardial activity. Direct myocardial depression occurs, in addition to an increase in vagal activity. The rate of oxygen transfer in between the contractions may not be sufficient to maintain adequate oxygenation, which will be characterised by a decrease, or absence, of variability and, eventually, baseline tachycardia.

Causes. Any condition which causes a reduction in placental blood flow may result in late decelerations, for example:

Placental abruption
Maternal hypotension
Excessive uterine activity.

In addition, any maternal or pregnancy-related disease which may result in placental pathology can also cause late decelerations, for example:

Diabetes mellitus
Pregnancy-induced hypertension
Renal disease.

Any fetus that is already compromised, either by lack of stored glycogen, or a reduction in circulating red blood cells for the transfer of oxygen, is also at an increased risk of developing late decelerations.

Examples of such predisposing circumstances are:

Intrauterine growth retardation
Prematurity
Rhesus isoimmunisation
Twin-to-twin transfusion.

Late decelerations are always associated with significant fetal hypoxia.

Management. The aim is to increase the uterine blood flow and oxygen transfer across the placenta to the fetus.

1. Change maternal posture.
2. Increase or commence intravenous infusion.
3. Give facial oxygen.
4. Stop any oxytocic infusion if in progress.

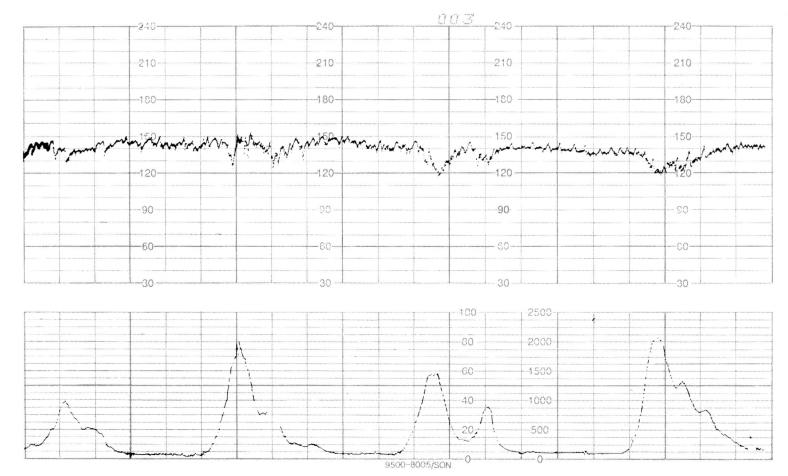

Fig. 2.3 *Early decelerations.*

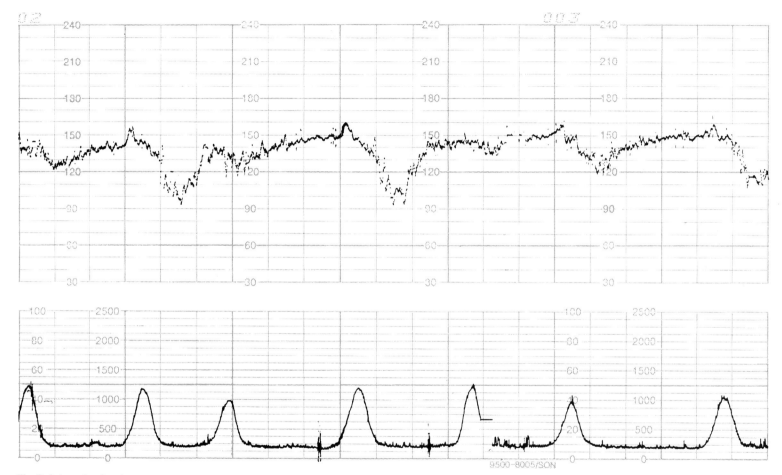

Fig. 2.4 *Late decelerations.*

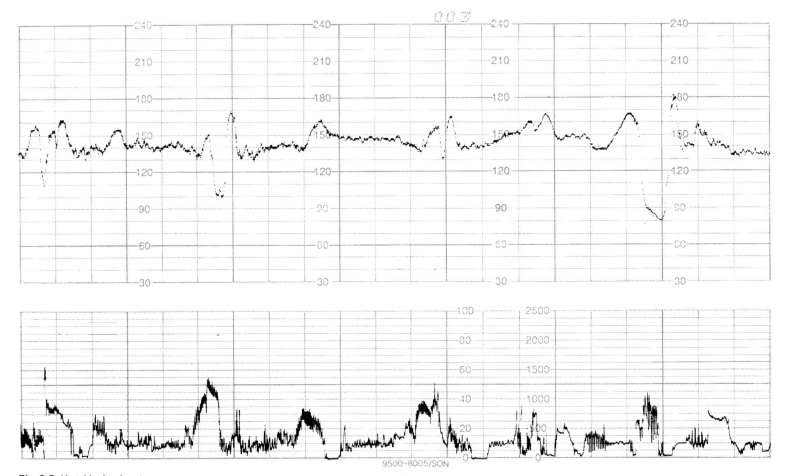

Fig. 2.5 *Variable decelerations.*

5. A fetal blood sample should be obtained to assess the pH value and base excess of the fetal blood.
6. Whilst the above actions are being undertaken, the mother should be prepared for delivery, particularly if the variability is decreased or if baseline tachycardia or bradycardia develops in between the decelerations.

Variable decelerations

Definition. Variable decelerations are inconsistent in shape and in their relationship to uterine contractions. They tend to have an amplitude of 40 b.p.m. or more. Accelerations often precede and follow the contraction. Variable decelerations are often mistakenly identified as early, however the physiological cause and subsequent management is different so care must be taken. It should be remembered that early decelerations are relatively uncommon, if diagnosing them think twice and check the criteria.

Figure 2.5 shows an example CTG exhibiting variable decelerations.

Aetiology. Variable decelerations appear to occur as the result of transient compression of the umbilical cord, between the fetus and surrounding maternal tissues or fetal parts, during a uterine contraction.

During a uterine contraction, the venous return is obstructed, leading to a decrease in venous return to the fetal heart. This in turn results in a decrease in cardiac output, and therefore arterial pressure. The baroreceptors in the aortic arch are stimulated and sympathetic activity is increased, resulting in a rise in the fetal heart rate to maintain the blood pressure. With further cord compression, the arterial flow becomes obstructed and fetal hypertension results. The baroreceptors in the aortic arch are stimulated, this time resulting in increased parasympathetic activity leading to a fall in the fetal heart rate, also in an attempt to maintain the blood pressure at a normal level. The deceleration now occurs. As the contraction subsides and the arterial flow obstruction is removed, fetal hypotension recurs until the venous flow returns to normal. A reactionary tachycardia develops. When the contraction has ended, the venous flow returns to normal and the fetal heart rate returns to the baseline.

The effect of variable decelerations upon the fetus varies depending upon the duration and degree of cord occlusion that occurs during a contraction. The longer that the deceleration lasts, and the greater the amplitude, the more suggestive it is of fetal compromise. However, the baseline of the fetal heart and the variability in between the decelerations are the best indicators of fetal oxygenation.

Causes. Variable decelerations are commonly seen when there is any form of umbilical cord entanglement, for example:

Umbilical cord around the neck or body
True knot in the umbilical cord
Prolapsed umbilical cord.

Management. This is aimed at attempting to relieve the cord compression:

1. Change the maternal posture.
2. Vaginal examination to exclude cord prolapse if this is deemed to be a possibility.
3. Stop any oxytocic infusion, if in progress.
4. Increase intravenous fluids.
5. Give facial oxygen.
6. If the decelerations are persistent, severe, or if the variability in between them is reduced, fetal blood sampling should be performed to assess the pH value and base excess of the blood. The mother should be prepared for delivery while this is being performed.

Prolonged deceleration

Definition. A prolonged deceleration is described as consisting of a drop in the fetal heart rate of 30 b.p.m. or more, lasting for a period of at least 2 minutes (for an example CTG, see Fig. 2.6).

Aetiology. Prolonged decelerations are caused by a decrease in oxygen transfer across the placenta to the fetus, usually as a result of a decrease in uterine blood flow. The chemoreceptors in the aortic arch are stimulated, resulting in an increase in parasympathetic activity and a fall in the fetal heart rate.

Prolonged decelerations are commonly associated with preceding variable decelerations.

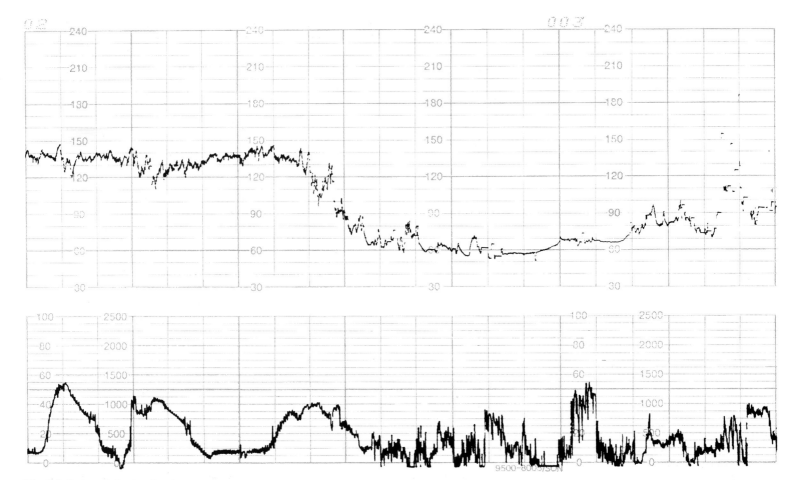

Fig. 2.6 *Prolonged decelerations.*

Causes

1. Total umbilical cord occlusion, e.g. cord prolapse.
2. Maternal hypotension resulting from the administration of local anaesthetic via an epidural catheter.
3. Uterine hypertonia.
4. Prolonged decelerations can also be evident following vaginal examination or artificial rupture of the membranes. This could be due to direct pressure being applied onto the fetal head, resulting in pressure on the vagal centre in the brain.

Management. This is aimed at increasing the blood flow to the uterus, and the oxygen transfer across the placenta to the fetus in addition to ascertaining the cause of the deceleration:

1. Change the maternal posture.
2. Increase intravenous fluids.
3. Stop oxytocic infusion, if in progress.
4. Give facial oxygen.
5. Vaginal examination to exclude cord prolapse.
6. Assess maternal blood pressure, particularly if an epidural block is in progress.
7. Prepare the mother for delivery while the above actions are being performed.
8. Obtain a fetal blood sample on recovery of the fetal heart rate to the baseline to assess the pH value and base excess of the blood. If this is performed during the deceleration, then a transient acidosis will be present, but may not be a true reflection of the degree of fetal hypoxia.

If the CTG has been normal beforehand, a definite cause can be attributed to the deceleration, appropriate management is initiated and the fetal heart rate returns to normal, the fetal outcome is usually good. If the variability is decreased, or any other fetal heart rate abnormalities are present, then this is more suggestive of significant fetal hypoxia.

MANAGEMENT OF FETAL HEART RATE ABNORMALITIES

The management of the periodic changes in the fetal heart rate that have been suggested are aimed at reducing the degree of fetal hypoxia and therefore improving the CTG. The measures, excluding fetal blood sampling, are non-invasive and can be performed quickly.

Medical staff should be informed of any fetal heart rate abnormalities that occur on a CTG. The actions suggested can be performed while waiting for them to attend, in the hope that an improvement in the pattern will be evident before they arrive.

Many single fetal heart rate abnormalities will resolve with conservative management (Grant 1989). In cases where multiple abnormalities are evident, conservative management, whilst preparations are being made to expedite delivery, may not greatly improve the degree of fetal hypoxia.

If the cause of the fetal heart rate abnormality can be ascertained, e.g. late decelerations occurring due to overstimulation of uterine activity with an oxytocic infusion, and the stimulus removed, the fetus is likely to recover more quickly in utero than if it were delivered in a severely hypoxic condition (Cohen & Schifrin 1978).

Attempts should always be made to employ conservative management of fetal heart rate abnormalities, even if a decision has been made to deliver the fetus immediately.

FETAL COMPROMISE

Fetal compromise occurs as a result of an asphyxial insult which gives rise to intrauterine hypoxia. Fetal heart rate abnormalities on a CTG should alert staff to the possibility that some degree of hypoxia exists (Arulkumaran & Chua 1996). Fetal hypoxia develops when insufficient oxygen is transferred from the mother to the fetus through the placenta, or if the transfer of oxygen is adequate, but the fetus is unable to utilise it owing to, for example, impaired circulation.

Throughout pregnancy, the fetus depends upon supplies of glucose and oxygen from the mother, which are necessary for its energy requirements. Some of the glucose is utilised immediately, the remainder being stored in the liver as glycogen, particularly during the third trimester of pregnancy. During labour, when maternal supplies of glucose and oxygen are diminished, and energy requirements raised, the fetus can draw upon these reserves of glycogen. The fetus converts the stored glycogen into acids; then, in the presence of oxygen, into carbon dioxide and water. The carbon dioxide is rapidly disposed of by diffusion across the placenta. This process requires blood flow to be effective. If there is any impairment, i.e. umbilical cord occlusion or placental abruption, the transfer of oxygen and carbon dioxide between the mother and fetus is diminished. This results in a rise in the carbon dioxide levels in the blood of the fetus. Carbonic acid is formed by the hydration of the excess carbon dioxide. Subsequently, a respiratory acidosis develops. The pH value of the blood falls, i.e. becomes more acid, although little change is seen in the acid–base balance or base excess, suggesting that the buffers that exist in the blood to neutralise acids and maintain the pH are still in evidence.

Respiratory acidosis can arise quickly and can also recover quickly if adequate oxygenation is resumed. This involves increasing the uterine blood flow and therefore the rate of transfer of oxygen and carbon dioxide across the placenta.

If respiratory acidosis is not corrected, and the transfer of oxygen to the fetus from the mother is not improved, then insufficient

oxygen is available to convert the acids, produced in the metabolism of glycogen, into carbon dioxide and water. The fetus is only able to dispose of these acids by diffusion through the placenta, which is a much slower process than the diffusion of carbon dioxide. Levels of lactic acid accumulate in the fetal circulation, resulting in a metabolic acidosis. The pH value of the blood falls, becoming more acidic, while the acid–base balance or base excess rises, suggesting that the buffers of the blood are being utilised rapidly in an attempt to maintain the pH. The presence of a metabolic acidosis implies that the length and severity of the asphyxial insult that has resulted in hypoxia has been more prolonged than the presence of a respiratory acidosis suggests.

Under normal circumstances, adequate oxygenation of the fetal tissues is maintained by the good uterine blood flow, the high fetal cardiac output and the enhanced oxygen-carrying capacity of the fetal blood. However, in circumstances where the placenta does not function adequately, or placental pathology develops, fetal oxygenation may be impaired, for example in:

Diabetes mellitus
Pregnancy-induced hypertension
Placental abruption
Postmaturity.

The fetus's ability to compensate for hypoxia is also impaired if the glycogen stores are reduced. The fetus is then unable to create

sufficient energy from the metabolism of the stores. Examples of such circumstances are:

Prematurity
Intrauterine growth retardation.

Any condition present in the fetus that involves a reduction in the oxygen-carrying capacity of the blood will also lead to a predisposition to developing hypoxia, for example:

Anaemia
Rhesus incompatibility
Twin-to-twin transfusion
Fetal infection when oxygen requirements are raised.

FETAL BLOOD SAMPLING

Fetal heart rate abnormalities arising on a CTG should be considered as an alerting factor to the possibility that the fetus is suffering some degree of hypoxia. However, this is a subjective diagnosis. For the diagnosis to be more accurate, interpretation of the CTG should be combined with fetal blood sampling, and the assessment of the pH value and base excess of the fetal blood. In 1985 MacDonald and colleagues concluded that there was little justification for the use of electronic fetal monitoring without the facilities to assess fetal acid–base status; a view supported by others (RCOG 1993, Murphy et al 1990, Van Den Berg et al 1987, Sawers 1983), and recommended by NICE (2001).

REFERENCES

Arulkumaran S, Chua S (1996) Cardiotocograph in labour. Current Obstetrics and Gynaecology 6(4): 182–188

Cohen W, Schifrin B (1978) Diagnosis and management of fetal distress during labour. Seminars in Perinatology 2(2): 155–167

Egley C C, Bowes W A Jr, Wagner D (1991) Sinusoidal fetal heart rate pattern during labour. American Journal of Perinatology 8: 197–202

Grant A (1989) Monitoring the fetus during labour. In: Chalmers I, Enkin M, Keirse M (eds) Effective care in pregnancy and childbirth. Oxford University Press, Oxford, p 846–888

MacDonald D, Grant A, Sheridan-Pereira M, Boylen P, Chalmers I (1985) The Dublin randomised controlled trial of intrapartum fetal heart rate monitoring. American Journal of Obstetrics and Gynecology 52: 524–539

Murphy K W, Johnston P, Moorcraft J (1990) Birth asphyxia and the intrapartum cardiotocograph. British Journal of Obstetrics and Gynaecology 97(6): 470–479

NICE (2001) The use of electronic fetal monitoring. Inherited Clinical Guideline C. NICE, London

O'Connor M C, Hassabo M S, McFadyen R (1980) Is the sinusoidal fetal heart rate pattern sinister? Journal of Obstetrics and Gynaecology. 1(2): 90–95

RCOG (Royal College of Obstetricians and Gynaecologists) (1993) Twenty Sixth RCOG Study Group. Intrapartum fetal surveillance. RCOG Press, London

Sawers R S (1983) Fetal monitoring during labour. British Medical Journal 287 (6406): 1649–1650

Van Den Berg P, Schmidt S, Gesch J (1987) Fetal distress and the condition of the newborn using cardiotocography and fetal blood analysis during labour. British Journal of Obstetrics and Gynaecology 94(1): 72–75

Young B K, Katz M, Wilson S J (1980) Sinusoidal fetal heart rate. Clinical significance. American Journal of Obstetrics and Gynecology 136: 587–593

RECOMMENDED RESOURCES

Enkin M, Keirse M J N C, Renfrew M, Neilson J (eds) (1996) Care of the fetus during labour. In: A guide to effective care in pregnancy and childbirth. Oxford University Press, Oxford, ch 30
An excellent resource containing a collection and systematic review of randomised trials in obstetric and midwifery practice. Each chapter ends with a comment by the reviewer on the implications for practice. Also available in an electronic database, The Cochrane Library, updated as reviews occur (see below).

Gibb D, Arulkamaran S (1997) Fetal monitoring in practice, 2nd edn. Butterworth Heinemann, Oxford
Clear and concise book on fetal well being, heart rate monitoring and techniques. There are helpful explanations of monitoring techniques with illustrations. There is also an exposition of trace analysis with examples offered.

MIDIRS (Midwives Information and Resource Service) and the NHS Centre for Reviews and Dissemination
- Fetal heart rate monitoring in labour. Informed choice for professionals leaflet
- Listening to your baby's heartbeat during labour. Informed choice for mothers leaflet. MIDIRS, Bristol

These leaflets are based on the best scientific evidence available. There are two leaflets for each topic, one for the professional and one for the mother. Clear, easy to read.

The Cochrane Library, Update Software, Oxford
This is an electronic database of systematic reviews updated as new trials are reported and gives the best available evidence in a number of areas including childbirth. Published in CD-ROM or disk format. Most maternity units have this database which is accessible by midwives and doctors.

PART 3

Litigation and risk management

Andrew Symon

INTRODUCTION

This chapter places the importance of cardiotocography (CTG) within its legal context by examining the relevant literature and using a number of legal cases to illustrate critical areas. It then identifies how risk management tries to reduce the incidence of poor clinical outcomes through encouraging appropriate training and supervision for those who use the CTG, and through its judicious use.

Risk management in health care is a wide concept, covering many different fields, including clinical competence, and the health and safety of all who enter a hospital. This chapter is only concerned with one very specific aspect of risk management, namely the use of the CTG and its relationship with litigation.

CTG is an aspect of clinical care which has attracted considerable attention in legal cases, particularly those concerning cerebral palsy. While its level of use may be debated, those doctors and midwives who use this form of monitoring must be adequately trained in its interpretation. Designed as a means of identifying the compromised fetus, the CTG has obvious clinical (as well as medico-legal) implications. Nevertheless, its routine application has been criticised.

BACKGROUND

Electronic fetal monitoring was pioneered in 1958 by Hon, but the first commercially available monitor was not produced until 1968 (Gibb & Arulkumaran 1997). Since that time CTG use has grown rapidly (some would say uncritically), although in recent years there has been more of a debate about when its use is most appropriate (see end of this section).

Fourteen years ago Murphy et al (1990, p. 38) claimed that continuous monitoring had become integral to obstetric practice, 'despite the fact that no clear evidence exists for its efficacy, especially in low risk pregnancy'. Their study found a low degree of specificity (i.e. many false positives — staff diagnosing fetal compromise when it did not exist) and they concluded that this was one of the main reasons for current dissatisfaction with this method of monitoring. They stressed the need to view the CTG in conjunction with other assessments (such as fetal blood sampling (FBS)), and not as the sole indicator of the fetal condition, a claim repeated more recently by Steer (1999). Despite this, the use of FBS varies enormously, and there has been a tendency among some practitioners to consider the CTG in isolation.

It must be remembered that the CTG is only one marker of possible fetal compromise: its ability to identify with certainty the compromised fetus and so prevent birth asphyxia is therefore limited. The term 'birth asphyxia' is one which, while frequently used, is defined in many different ways. There is no way of measuring asphyxia directly (i.e. measuring oxygen levels on the brain at cellular level), and so indirect measures or markers are used. These include the CTG, fetal or cord blood pH, or a baby's condition at birth (assessed by the Apgar score) or neurological status in the first few days of life.

The particular clinical (as well as legal) concern in monitoring a labour is to prevent the hypoxia which can cause damage to brain cells leading to handicap or even death. The condition which has attracted the most attention in this respect is cerebral palsy. Nearly twenty years ago Hensleigh et al (1986, p. 979) noted that 'the incidence of cerebral palsy in developed countries is about 1.5 to 2.5 per 1000. Comparisons between countries show no correlation with the prevailing perinatal mortality rate'. In other words, intrapartum monitoring measures which were designed to reduce perinatal mortality will have little impact on the incidence of cerebral palsy, since the factors leading to the two outcomes are apparently different. Ten years ago Stanley (1994) noted that obstetric technology had done nothing to reduce the incidence of cerebral palsy — indeed, it had increased slightly, a factor attributed to the survival of low birth weight babies who would probably not have survived twenty or thirty years ago (Colver et al 2000).

An international consensus statement on the link between intrapartum events and cerebral palsy (MacLennan 1999, p. 1055) noted that 'a large proportion of cases are associated with maternal or antenatal factors such as prematurity, intrauterine growth restriction, intrauterine infection, fetal coagulation disorders, multiple pregnancy, antepartum haemorrhage, breech presentation, and chromosomal or congenital anomalies'.

Given this apparently limited ability to influence overall cerebral palsy rates, the CTG must be used with caution: it is not a panacea for the problem of handicapped infants. When it is used, it must be used for the right reason, and with the appropriate degree of skill. However, some studies have demonstrated considerable difficulties with interpretation of the CTG, including a high degree of false positives and false negatives (Keegan et al 1985), high levels of confidence in the ability to interpret CTGs, even amongst those midwives who spend little time in the labour ward (Stewart & Guildea 2002), and differences not only between practitioners (Henderson-Smart 1991), but also when the same practitioner examines the same trace twice (Nielsen et al 1987). The RCOG Clinical Guideline on the use of electronic fetal monitoring (RCOG 2001) reported that a greater emphasis on education and training appeared to improve knowledge levels and could improve clinical skills. However, it noted that there was insufficient evidence to conclude that one training format (e.g. lectures, computer-assisted sessions) was more effective than another (cf. Wilson & Mires 2000). An abbreviated

guideline based on the full RCOG paper was published by NICE (see RCOG 2001).

There is a recognition that blanket CTG use is inappropriate. The RCOG Clinical Guideline (RCOG 2001, p. 17) recommends that continuous monitoring 'should be offered and recommended for high-risk pregnancies where there is an increased risk of perinatal death, cerebral palsy, or neonatal encephalopathy' and 'where oxytocin is being used for induction or augmentation of labour'. Williams and Arulkumaran (2004, p. 458) note that 'the CTG ... is helpful in identifying asphyxiating conditions during labour in a small group of babies at risk of death or irreversible brain injury'.

This more targeted approach to electronic fetal monitoring is to be welcomed, and will be seen in medico-legal considerations. A midwife's actions are judged by whether she acted appropriately in a given situation, e.g. did she initiate CTG monitoring when she should have done? With more specific use, and better education and training regarding its use and interpretation, it is to be hoped that some of the legal problems encountered in the past will become more rare. Successive confidential enquiries into stillbirths and deaths in infancy (e.g. MCHRC 1997, 1998) have highlighted the CTG as a significant factor in poor outcomes. Other studies have identified staff deficiencies in CTG use which have resulted in litigation (Symon 2001, James 1991, Vincent et al 1991, Capstick & Edwards 1990, Ennis & Vincent 1990)

THE CTG IN LITIGATION

The law regarding clinical negligence is ably covered in standard texts (e.g. Montgomery 2003, Dimond 2002) and I do not propose to cover this. Similarly, it is beyond the scope of this chapter to discuss the possible motives behind litigation, or the likelihood of success when people do sue. Such issues, among others, are considered elsewhere (Symon 2001). The object here is to demonstrate how the CTG features in litigation.

In the early 1990s there was a flurry of interest in obstetric litigation. A number of small-scale studies highlighted various aspects of this topic, and these are briefly reviewed here. These studies, in describing patterns of litigation, raised concerns about the efficiency and expense of the legal system when dealing with medical negligence claims, and so helped to pave the way for legal reforms. Lord Woolf's Access to Justice (Woolf 1996) report aimed to make the system more equitable for all concerned. However, the National Audit Office's report into clinical negligence found that almost £4 bn would be needed to meet the cost of known and anticipated NHS claims (NAO 2001). This led to suggestions that no-fault schemes and structured settlements should be introduced, along with greater use of alternative methods of dispute resolution, such as mediation.

The Lord Chancellor's recent report (LCD 2002) has highlighted the political desire for further reform: litigation is to be avoided where possible, and less complex and less adversarial when it does occur. The time and money spent on cases is to be reduced, partly through employing judges more effectively. To understand how we have arrived at this situation, it is necessary to explain some of the history of recent obstetric litigation, and in particular the place of CTG within this subject.

Ennis and Vincent's (1990) study of 64 obstetric legal cases found a number of complaints made about CTGs. These included unsatisfactory or missing traces, abnormalities being ignored or not noticed, and traces simply not being done. Of eleven in this category, they note that in three 'midwives were asked by a doctor to carry out CTG but forgot' (Ennis & Vincent 1990, p. 1366). The problem of a CTG trace going missing was also noted by James (1991, p. 38): 'The cardiotocograph record is often crucial yet its bulk at the end of a long and complicated labour makes it difficult to store securely within the records. However, claims have become indefensible because this vital piece of evidence was missing, the notes were inadequate, or key personnel could not be traced'.

Capstick and Edwards (1990) identified problems with not noticing signs of fetal distress, or not taking appropriate action quickly when such signs were noticed. Vincent et al (1991, p. 392) noted that missing or poor quality traces were significant, and also found

that interpretation was a recurrent theme: 'In 14 cases the doctor or midwife simply did not recognise an abnormal trace. In five the abnormality was noted, but no action was taken; the staff believed the machine to be faulty and so ignored the trace'.

These features all point to significant deficiencies in staff competence, whether they relate to clinical abilities or communication skills. Such deficiencies have also been highlighted in cases reported in risk management and legal journals (see list of legal cases at the end). The various features highlighted in these claims were in evidence in many of the cases which formed part of my own large-scale study into perinatal litigation*. A small selection of these cases is reported here. I have used extracts to illustrate some of the circumstances in which the CTG has become integral to a legal action. These include failing to use the CTG when there is an indication to do so, the inappropriate use of equipment and poor interpretation of the CTG trace. These extracts are merely illustrative,

---

*The legal cases referred to have not, to my knowledge, been reported in legal or other journals. They come from Scotland and England, and were examined during the course of doctoral research based at the University of Edinburgh, 1993–1997. Funding and support for this came from the Economic and Social Research Council, the National Board for Nursing, Midwifery and Health Visiting for Scotland, the Iolanthe Research Fellowship, and Perth and Kinross Healthcare NHS Trust.

and the success (or otherwise) of these cases should not be inferred from the brief extracts given.

One point well worth making is that legal cases involving cerebral palsy often are not raised for several years, and may take many years to be resolved (Symon 2002). This may cause significant distress for practitioners and parents alike. It is in everyone's interests to minimise the incidence of such litigation.

When to monitor?

In one of the cases reviewed, there were persistent early fetal heart rate (FHR) decelerations. The midwifery staff appeared to think these were benign, despite there being reduced FHR variability and meconium staining of the liquor. The expert report stated:

> *Case 1* 'There is a period of 90 minutes … when there was no CTG recording. This is an unacceptable situation where the patient has had a previous section, (is) at 42 weeks with meconium staining, and with CTG abnormalities which are persistent and who was on Oxytocin.'

This catalogue of 'at risk' factors does not appear to have alerted midwives to the need for extra vigilance, and unsurprisingly this case was conceded by the defence. However, given the desire of some pregnant women for minimal monitoring and intervention in labour, the decision to use the CTG is evidently not always automatic, even when certain 'at risk' factors are present. In another case the woman complained that she should have been monitored more closely, despite having asked in advance of her labour for minimal monitoring. In fact during labour the CTG had been discontinued at her request due to discomfort. Her solicitor claimed:

> Case 2 'Continuous fetal monitoring when the decision was made to give a syntocinon infusion should have been insisted upon …'

While many staff would agree that the use of Syntocinon (oxytocin) to augment labour is an indication for continuous monitoring by CTG (and it is now recommended in the RCOG guideline), this case illustrates the balancing act which staff must attempt. On the one hand there is a desire to accede to a specific request, and on the other using clinical judgement and (increasingly) following unit protocols which may contradict the woman's stated preference. Sadly, cases involving the use (and misuse) of Syntocinon (oxytocin) are not rare. In addition to careful monitoring and sympathetic care, midwives must keep meticulous notes in this situation, and this includes a full account of the nature of the uterine contractions.

Difficulties with monitoring
Midwives have sometimes found it difficult to monitor effectively:

> Case 3 The plaintiffs claimed that monitoring should not have been discontinued. The

midwife documented that it was very difficult to listen to the fetal heart as the labouring woman moved and rocked a lot.

The midwife looking after her noted frequent 'loss of contact' on the CTG trace, and stated: 'I made the decision to stop the print out from the monitor but kept the transducer and belt in situ, and I was continually listening to the fetal heart'.

The midwives' reports indicated that the fetal heart rate was satisfactory at all times, but there is clearly a difficulty in situations like this. When a probe must be held in position in order to hear the fetal heart rate clearly, writing contemporaneous entries in the woman's case notes is impossible. In another case the midwife stated:

> Case 4 'As I was anxious to get a better quality CTG, I didn't take my hands off the transducer and was aware that I wasn't recording this in the case notes.'

The CTG tracing must be of sufficient quality that others can interpret it. Williams and Arulkumaran (2004, p. 459) note: 'The Courts will view an uninterpretable CTG with utmost suspicion and such a recording might jeopardise a successful defence'. The midwife must be able to ensure several things at once: in addition to the clinical care she gives the labouring woman, she must make sure that a reasonable CTG trace is produced, and that she

completes the clinical notes as soon as she can. It may be that having notepaper to hand, and writing times and heart rates down as an 'aide-mémoire' would help.

Using the equipment correctly
In another legal case the plaintiff's solicitors claimed:

> Case 5 'It would appear that a foetal monitor was incorrectly adjusted and, accordingly, the readings which it gave were not properly interpreted and significant abnormalities were disregarded.'

The CTG had 'wrong speed' written on it. It transpired that different speeds were used at different times in labour, and no times were logged, so the trace was more difficult to interpret. (The case occurred a number of years ago; more modern CTG machines automatically print the date and time on the trace regularly.)

There have been times when the CTG machine itself appears to cause problems:

> Case 6 The plaintiff's solicitors claimed that instead of diagnosing fetal distress in labour, staff assumed the 'heart rate coming and going' was due to a defective CTG machine. Only when the third machine (they claim) was showing the same sort of trace was the woman sent for caesarean section.

There was nothing documented to say the CTG machine was replaced at all.

Eventually the CTG traces were found, and they revealed one change of machine, from an old to a new model.

The fact that equipment is defective is no defence. In this case there was a gap of 2½ hours when the CTG was not on. There were six written recordings of a fetal heart rate during this period, at half-hourly intervals. The expert report criticised the midwives for not having a more detailed record. Documentation is discussed in the Risk Management section.

Interpretation of the trace

It seems obvious to state that staff who use CTGs must be able to interpret them, but sadly this ability is lacking all too often. Williams and Arulkumaran (2004, p. 460) claim that 'CTG misinterpretation is the most common source of alleged negligence in obstetric litigation and the inexact nature of CTG traces causes great confusion in Court'. In one case the expert report stated:

> Case 5 'I do not recall having ever seen a trace with such a smooth line and almost complete lack of beat to beat variation … The nursing (sic) staff faithfully recorded the events but apparently failed to appreciate the significance of the flat trace and therefore did not report it to the medical staff.'

There are other cases in which the CTG has shown abnormalities which were ignored by staff. In one instance the expert reported:

Case 7 'It is difficult to see the point of fetal monitoring if no action is to be taken when there are obvious abnormalities in the recording.'

Staff must be educated and trained in order to make an intelligent interpretation of CTG traces. However, all too frequently it must be questioned whether staff are adequately prepared for this part of their work. In another case a junior midwife was heavily criticised by the defence solicitor:

> Case 8 '(The midwife) admitted quite freely that she spent many hours in watching a fetal heart monitor which she was insufficiently trained to interpret or understand at the time. She has since been better trained and, looking back at the fetal heart traces during the period she was on duty, she sees them as being abnormal. In my opinion, quite a bit of liability must therefore attach to a system which asked midwives to watch a monitor which they are insufficiently trained to understand.'

All staff, of whatever grade, must be trained in CTG interpretation if they are called upon to use the technology, and it would appear that most units have taken this on board. In addition, practitioners must take the full clinical picture into account when interpreting the CTG, not just the information portrayed on the trace.

Delay in responding

A delay in appropriate management may result either from non-recognition of an abnormal trace, or inaction following the diagnosis of such an abnormality. Appropriate action may be to 'wait and see' for a limited period (e.g. while the Syntocinon (oxytocin) infusion is reduced or discontinued, or maternal hydration carried out) but this must be explained fully in the notes. Williams and Arulkumaran (2004, p. 460) state: 'Initialling the CTG is not enough'.

Ennis and Vincent (1990) report that in some of the legal cases they analysed midwives had correctly noted a fetal heart rate abnormality, but this was ignored by the doctor. Clearly there may be differences of opinion at times. Such differences were highlighted in related research (Symon 1998) which examined the views of a large number of midwives and obstetricians concerning litigation and certain related aspects. In this research one doctor commented that: 'Over diagnosis of "distress" is a large problem'.

From the midwife's point of view there came this comment: 'It can be very frustrating for midwives to inform doctors of a suspected abnormality, to have it ignored before the client, and to have to repeatedly call the doctor back'.

Such differences of opinion must be addressed, and it is one of the aims of risk management to do this. However, it is more concerning when a midwife fails to take appropriate steps to call in more senior colleagues, as in this case in which a consultant obstetrician reported:

> Case 9 'There is little doubt that at 23.30 hours acute profound fetal bradycardia occurred and the delay of 20 minutes before medical assistance was summoned is indefensible ... Equally it seems that the outcome was not helped by the six minute interval between delivery and the arrival of the paediatrician ... What is inexcusable is that he was not summoned prior to the delivery given the circumstances of this profound and protracted bradycardia in the last half hour of labour.'

Maternity care is multi-disciplinary, and midwives must appreciate the respective roles of other practitioners and involve them appropriately.

RISK MANAGEMENT

As stated in the introduction, risk management covers many different areas, even within maternity care. Although the previous section examined the role of the CTG in litigation, it should not be concluded that risk management aims only to minimise potential exposure to litigation, although this is of course one of its aims. The introduction of 'clinical governance', which is aimed at improving service quality and ensuring high standards, incorporated risk management as one of its tools. It is also worth pointing out that, in recent years, there has been a shift in focus away from conceptualising clinical errors as simply the result of individual fault. There is an increased recognition that poor outcomes often occur because of latent conditions within a unit which prepare the ground for mistakes (Reason 2001). While the systems-based approach to risk management acknowledges the role that underlying conditions may have in the process of poor outcomes, there is still a need to ensure that individual practitioners perform to a satisfactory standard at least.

Clinical risk management aims to minimise the incidence and impact of adverse outcomes, and to facilitate effective claims management through an early investigation and assessment of the event (Vincent & Walshe 2001). While there may be some debate as to what exactly constitutes an adverse outcome, it is clear that the perception of the women concerned (and possibly that of her family) is crucial. There is a considerable literature about expectations and experiences. Some of this describes the belief that health service practitioners have contributed to high (and sometimes unrealistic) expectations and to consequent dissatisfaction with a less than ideal outcome (cf. Wilson & Symon 2002, Symon 1998, Ranjan 1993).

Within obstetrics and midwifery — and in terms of risk management we must acknowledge that perinatal care is a multi-disciplinary field — there are several areas that can be targeted from a risk management point of view. Effective teamwork and inter-disciplinary communication is essential (Firth-Cozens 2001). Documentation is also a critical area: without a detailed (and legible) account of the events in question it may be impossible to determine whether a particular outcome may have been prevented, and whether the appropriate lessons will be learned.

Training and supervision

It is essential that staff who are called upon to interpret CTG traces are competent to do so. In-service education is the standard means of ensuring this but it was worrying to find in a large-scale survey of obstetricians and midwives (Symon 1998) that 65% of the obstetricians felt that training for midwives was deficient in this regard and that many midwives agreed with this. This must be a matter for concern, for it is the midwife who will usually first pick up on possible problems. The legal (and emotional) consequences of failing to do so may be devastating.

The RCOG guideline recommends 'annual training with assessment to ensure that ... skills are kept up to date' (RCOG 2001, p. 22). This is a minimum requirement: if attendance at a fire lecture can be mandatory in an attempt to reduce risk, then regular in-service training and education sessions on CTG use and interpretation must be mandatory for practitioners who use this technology. Differences of opinion over interpretation will continue to occur, but can be reduced by the thorough education of staff regarding the use *and limitations* of the CTG. As discussed in the Background section at the beginning of this chapter, the CTG is only one marker of the fetal condition.

With regard to competence, the NMC Code of Professional Conduct states: 'You must acknowledge the limits of your professional competence and only undertake practice and accept responsibilities for those activities in which you are competent' (NMC 2002, p. 8). While employers have a duty to provide training for their staff, individual midwives also have a responsibility to ensure that they are adequately prepared for the duties entrusted to them, and to request supervision where necessary.

New staff — especially newly-qualified staff — must be supervised until their competence is assured (Case 8 above makes this point). Competence cannot be assumed simply because someone has been in post for a few weeks or months. In this regard locum or agency staff present a particular problem: although qualified, their competence and skill may not have been demonstrated in that particular unit.

Communication

Drife (2001, p. 77) notes that 'The relationship between obstetricians and midwives has not always been easy', but claims that a spirit of co-operation existed by the end of the 1990s (he cites Towards Safer Childbirth as an example of this). The change in the Midwives' Rules which allowed midwives to call for help from an appropriately experienced midwifery colleague rather than being required to call a doctor (who may have been less experienced than the midwife), suggests greater mutual respect. If midwives are competent in interpreting CTG traces, but cannot (for whatever reason) communicate this either to a more senior midwife or a member of the medical staff, then there is a problem. Drife (2001, p. 91) suggests team-building social occasions and regular delivery suite meetings. The level of formality of such meetings may vary, but must at all costs avoid becoming a 'finger-pointing' exercise: that would destroy any hope of the mutual respect which underpins effective communication.

Communication between staff and the labouring woman, and (where appropriate, her family) is vital too: Dillner (1995) notes the role of poor communication in suboptimal outcomes. Monitoring can only be carried out with her consent, and this may be difficult to obtain if she is in pain or upset because of events, or is under the effects of opiate or inhalational analgesia.

Equipment

While it may be tempting to assume that equipment within maternity units is efficient and well-maintained, in view of the legal cases concerning apparently defective machinery, this is not a safe assumption. Obsolete monitors must be replaced, and those which are used maintained to an acceptable standard. This of course has cost implications, but must be more financially appealing than the prospect of paying out hundreds of thousands of pounds because monitoring was either deficient or not carried out at all.

Because the CTG is only one marker of the fetal condition, it is recommended that equipment for fetal blood sampling also be provided (Drife 2001, Steer 1999).

Documentation

This aspect of care has been highlighted by many authors (e.g. McRae 1999, James 1991), especially with regard to potential litigation. Cohn (1984, p. 321) notes that 'good record keeping is the single most useful thing that can be done to minimize risk, other than to talk with and take good care of patients'. Sadly, that very sensible advice from twenty years ago still needs to be reiterated today.

The CTG trace is part of the clinical documentation, and is therefore a legal document. The labouring woman's identification details must be recorded clearly on each trace. If the paper needs to be changed, then each section must be labelled so that the full trace can be reviewed in the correct order (Williams & Arulkumaran 2004).

The maternal pulse should be identified and recorded in the case notes so that there is no doubt as to whether the fetal heart rate or maternal pulse has been detected. This may happen if the abdominal transducer slips and has to be repositioned.

Because missing or deficient CTG traces have been a particular problem in litigation, it is vital that midwives also record the fetal heart rate in the woman's case notes. Entries relating to rate and variability, as well as accelerations and decelerations, will help to clarify the record of this important marker of the fetal condition in the event that the CTG trace is unavailable. These entries should be made in the notes as soon as possible: any delay decreases the likelihood that staff will be able to recall accurately a sequence of events and results. Failing to make any entries for long periods can leave the impression that the woman was unsupervised (not an uncommon allegation), and can give the impression that care was substandard. This is best summed up by the adage 'If you didn't write it, you didn't do it'. Of course, a balance must be struck: first and foremost a midwife must provide adequate care, but she must also ensure that an accurate record is made of this care.

However, a particular difficulty with the CTG is storage. Although we are likely to see increased electronic storage of CTG data in the next few years, most units will continue to use paper tracing for some time. Bear in mind that many legal actions are not raised for several years (in cases involving cerebral palsy there is effectively no time limit), and because the paper on which traces are printed is heat and light sensitive, and liable to tearing, it must be protected securely. Some units have introduced a sturdy envelope (for CTG traces only) which can be attached inside the case notes.

CONCLUSION

All the suggestions made here may seem obvious. However, to repeat a point made by Cohn (1984), if the problems caused by failing to implement these points were rare, they would not be cited here. Many poor outcomes (and subsequent legal cases) simply would not arise if these points were taken on board and implemented effectively. It is disheartening to realise that certain errors continue to be made despite a recognition that they can often be prevented. However, we don't live in an ideal world: staff will have 'off days', communication with colleagues and with women and their families may be difficult, and pressure of work may leave little time for writing in the case notes.

CTGs, however, remain a critical part of intrapartum care, and constitute a significant factor in litigation. Risk management in this respect is the responsibility both of employers and of individual practitioners. There is no magic wand which will make these problems go away, and while obvious, the suggestions for effective risk management require the support and co-operation of all grades of clinical staff and their managers.

REFERENCES

Capstick JB, Edwards P (1990) Trends in obstetric malpractice claims. Lancet 336: 931–2

Cohn S (1984) The nurse-midwife: malpractice and risk management. Journal of Nurse-Midwifery 29: 316–321

Colver AF, Gibson M, Hey EN et al (2000) Increasing rates of cerebral palsy across the severity spectrum in north-east England 1964–1993. The North of England Collaborative Cerebral Palsy Survey. Archives of Disease in Childhood (Fetal and Neonatal edition) 83(1): F7–F12

Dillner L (1995) Babies' deaths linked to suboptimal care. British Medical Journal 310: 757

Dimond B (2002) The legal aspects of midwifery, 2nd edn. Books for Midwives, Oxford

Drife JO (2001) Risk reduction in obstetrics. In: Vincent C (ed) Clinical risk management: enhancing patient safety, 2nd edn. BMJ Publishing Group, London

Ennis M, Vincent CA (1990) Obstetric accidents: a review of 64 cases. British Medical Journal 300: 1365–67

Firth-Cozens J (2001) Teams, culture, and managing risk. In: Vincent C (ed) Clinical risk management: enhancing patient safety 2nd edn. BMJ Publishing Group, London

Gibb D, Arulkumaran S (1997) Fetal monitoring in practice. Butterworth Heinemann, Oxford

Henderson-Smart D (1991) Throwing the baby out with the fetal monitoring? Medical Journal of Australia 154: 576–8

Hensleigh P, Fainstat T, Spencer R (1986) Perinatal events and cerebral palsy. American Journal of Obstetrics and Gynecology 154: 978–81

James C (1991) Risk Management in obstetrics and gynaecology. Journal of the Medical Defence Union 7: 36–38

Keegan K, Waffarn F, Quilligan E (1985) Obstetric characteristics and FHR patterns of infants during the newborn period. American Journal of Obstetrics and Gynecology 153: 732–7

LCD (Lord Chancellor's Department) (2002) Civil justice evaluation: further findings. The Lord Chancellor's Department.Online. Available: http://www.dca.gov.uk/civil/reform/ffreform.htm

MacLennan A (1999) A template for defining a causal relationship between acute intrapartum events and cerebral palsy: international consensus statement. British Medical Journal 319: 1054–59

MCHRC (Maternal and Child Health Research Consortium) (1997) Confidential enquiry into stillbirths and deaths in infancy. Sixth annual report. MCHRC, London

MCHRC (Maternal and Child Health Research Consortium) (1998) Confidential enquiry into stillbirths and deaths in infancy. Seventh annual report. MCHRC, London

McRae MJ (1999) Fetal surveillance and monitoring: legal issues revisited. Journal of Obstetric, Gynecologic and Neonatal Nursing 28(3): 310–9

Montgomery J (2003) Health care law, 2nd edn. OUP, Oxford

Murphy K, Johnson P, Moorcraft J et al (1990) Birth asphyxia and the intrapartum cardiotocograph. British Journal of Obstetrics and Gynaecology 97: 470–79

NAO (National Audit Office) (2001) Handling clinical negligence claims in England. HC 403. The Stationery Office, London

Nielsen P, Stigsby B, Nickelsen C et al (1987) Intra- and inter-observer variability in the assessment of intrapartum CTGs. Acta Obstetrica Gynecologica Scandinavica 66: 421–424

NMC (Nursing and Midwifery Council) (2002) Code of professional conduct. NMC, London

Ranjan V (1993) Obstetrics and the fear of litigation. Professional Care of Mother and Child January 1993: 10–12

RCOG (Royal College of Obstetricians and Gynaecologists) (2001) The use of electronic fetal monitoring: the use and interpretation of cardiotocography in intrapartum fetal surveillance. RCOG, London. Online. Available: (Full guideline) www.nice.org.uk/pdf/efmguidelinercog. pdf. (Abbreviated NICE guideline): www.nice.org.uk /pdf/efmguidelinenice.pdf

Reason J (2001) Understanding adverse events: the human factor. In: Vincent C (ed) Clinical risk management: enhancing patient safety 2nd edn. BMJ Publishing Group London

Stanley F (1994) Cerebral palsy — The courts catch up with sad realities. Medical Journal of Australia 161: 236

Steer P (1999) Assessment of mother and fetus in labour. British Medical Journal 318: 858–861

Stewart J, Guildea ZE (2002) Knowledge and skills of CTG interpretation. British Journal of Midwifery 10(8): 505–8

Symon A (1998) Who's accountable? Who's to blame? Litigation — the views of midwives and obstetricians. Hochland and Hochland, Hale

Symon A (2001) Obstetric litigation from A–Z. Quay Books, Salisbury

Symon A (2002) The significance of time factors in cerebral palsy litigation. Midwifery 18: 35–42

Vincent C, Martin T, Ennis M (1991) Obstetric accidents: the patient's perspective. British Journal of Obstetrics and Gynaecology 98: 390–395

Vincent C, Walshe K (2001) Clinical risk management and the analysis of clinical incidents. In: Clements RV (ed) Risk management and litigation in obstetrics and gynaecology. Royal Society of Medicine Press, London

Williams B, Arulkumaran S (2004) Cardiotocography and medicolegal issues. Best Practice and Research: Clinical Obstetrics and Gynaecology 18(3): 457–66

Wilson J, Symon A (eds) (2002) Clinical risk management in midwifery — the right to a perfect baby? Butterworth Heinemann, Oxford

Wilson T, Mires GJ (2000) A comparison of performance by medical and midwifery students in multiprofessional teaching. Medical Education 34(9): 744–6

Woolf (Lord) (1996) Access to justice. Final report by the Right Honourable the Lord Woolf, Master of the Rolls. HMSO, London

LEGAL CASES

These are just a selection of cases involving the CTG which have appeared in various legal and risk management journals over the years. Sadly, many more than these could have been included.

C v Norwich Health Authority (2003) Clinical Risk 9(2): 73–74

D v S Health Authority (2004) Health Care Risk Report May 6–7

Dowdie v Camberwell Health Authority (1997) 8 Medical Law Reports: 368–376

Dowson v Sunderland Hospitals NHS Trust (2004) Lloyd's Law Reports: Medical 177 (QBD)

E v Oxfordshire Health Authority (2002) Clinical Risk 8(3): 122–124

Gaughan v Bedfordshire Health Authority (1997) 8 Medical Law Reports: 182–190

Hockaday v Chester Health Authority (2003) Health Care Risk Report May 7–8

Jason Sean Berrell v Salford District Health Authority (2004). Health Care Risk Report April 8–9

Jenks v West Kent Health Authority (2001) Health Law 6(2): 4–5

K v Guy's & St Thomas' NHS Trust (2002) Clinical Risk 8(1): 40–41

KFB v Liverpool Health Authority (2003) Clinical Risk 9(3): 120–121

Lisle v Rochdale Healthcare NHS Trust (2002) Health Care Risk Report July 6–7

Miss X v North Staffordshire Health Authority (2004) Health Care Risk Report April 7–8

P v Preston Acute Hospitals NHS Trust (2002) Clinical Risk 8(3): 122

Robertson v Nottingham Health Authority (1997) 8 Medical Law Reports: 1–15

Smith-Tawiah v Northwick Park and St Mark's NHS Trust (2001) Health Law 6(6): 3–5

Trattles v Tees Health Authority (2003) Medical Litigation 2 Feb: 5–6

Wiszniewski v Central Manchester Health Authority (1996) 7 Medical Law Reports: 248–265

Wiszniewski v Central Manchester Health Authority (1998) Lloyd's Law Reports: Medical 223 (CA)

Case studies

CONTENTS

Normal

1

HISTORY

23-year-old gravida 2, para 0 + 1

Past history

Nil relevant

Antenatal period

Treated for urinary tract infection at 28 weeks
Admitted at 40 weeks with contractions

Labour

15.30 hours
Cervical os 2 cm dilated
Artificial rupture of membranes — clear liquor draining
Fetal scalp electrode applied
Intrauterine pressure catheter inserted
16.05 hours
Epidural analgesia commenced
17.45 hours
CTG (Fig. 4.1)

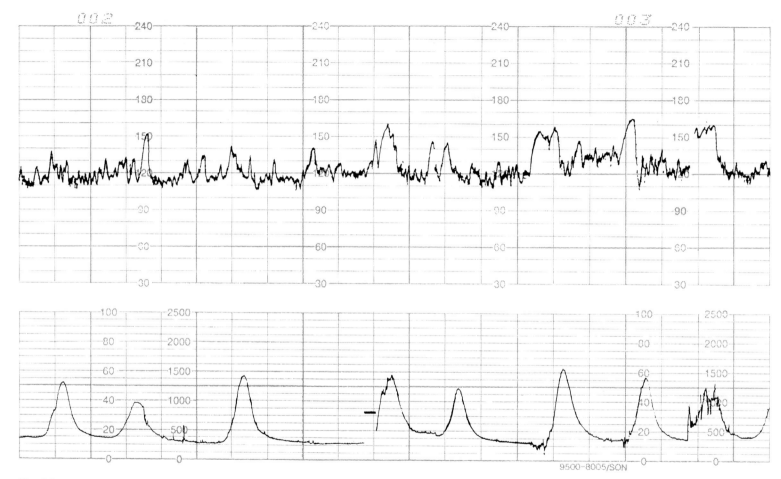

Fig. 4.1

CTG

1 What do you notice about the baseline?
2 What do you notice about the baseline variability?
3 What periodic changes, if any, are present?
4 What do you notice about the uterine activity?
5 What is the most probable cause of fetal heart rate abnormality shown on this trace?
6 What treatment and/or intervention would you consider necessary for this fetal heart rate pattern?

NOTES

1

2

3

4

5

6

ANALYSIS

1 Baseline 110–120 b.p.m.
2 Variability 5–10 b.p.m.
3 No decelerations, accelerations with some contractions
4 Contracting 4–5 in 10 minutes, varying in strength
5 Normal CTG
6 No action necessary

OUTCOME

04.00 hours
Progressed to second stage of labour
06.00 hours
No progress made
Caesarean section performed
Live boy
Apgar score 9/1 9/5
Birthweight 4.010 kg

2

25-year-old gravida 3, para 1 + 1

Past history
Nil relevant

Antenatal period
Twin pregnancy diagnosed on booking scan
Admitted at 37 weeks with spontaneous
rupture of membranes and contractions

Labour
04.00 hours
Cervical os 4 cm dilated
Clear liquor draining
Fetal scalp electrode applied to twin I (faint
line on CTG)
Twin II monitored externally (darker line on
CTG)
Contractions monitored externally
04.50 hours
Epidural analgesia commenced
06.00 hours
Cervical os 6 cm dilated
CTG (Fig. 4.2)

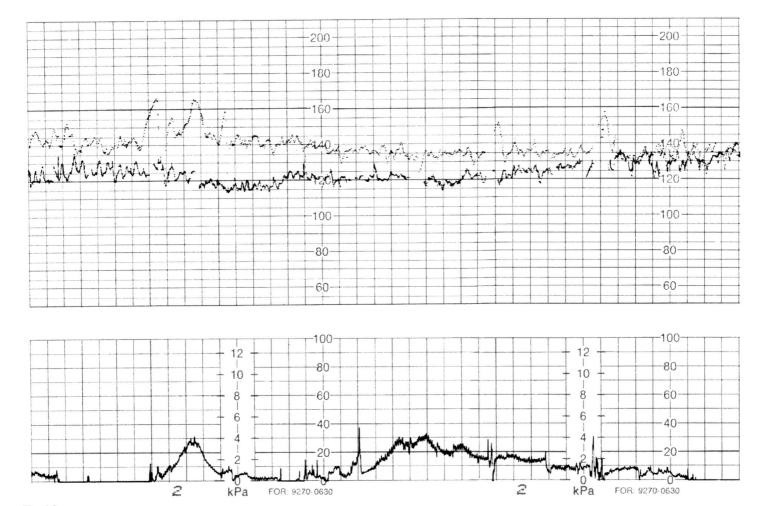

Fig. 4.2

CTG

1 What do you notice about the baseline?
2 What do you notice about the baseline variability?
3 What periodic changes, if any, are present?
4 What do you notice about the uterine activity?
5 What is the most probable cause of fetal heart rate abnormality shown on this trace?
6 What treatment and/or intervention would you consider necessary for this fetal heart rate pattern?

NOTES

1

2

3

4

5

6

ANALYSIS

1 Baseline
  Twin I: 130–145 b.p.m.
  Twin II: 115–120 b.p.m.
2 Variability
  Twin I: 5–10 b.p.m.
  Twin II: external, therefore not accurate;
  appears 5–10 beats.
3 No decelerations, accelerations present
4 Contractions not monitored adequately
5 Normal CTG
6 Contractions should be monitored
  No other action necessary

OUTCOME

10.35 hours
Progressed to second stage of labour
12.06 hours
Straight forceps delivery of twin I
Live girl
Apgar score 9/1 9/5
Birthweight 2.470 kg
12.20 hours
Straight forceps delivery of twin II
Live girl
Apgar score 8/1 9/5
Birthweight 2.560 kg

3

HISTORY

30-year-old gravida 2, para 1

Past history

Nil relevant

Antenatal period

Progressed normally
Admitted at 41 weeks plus 2 days' gestation in spontaneous labour

Labour

03.20 hours
Cervical os 7 cm dilated
Clear liquor draining
Requesting epidural analgesia
03.40 hours
Epidural analgesia commenced
Continuous external monitoring in progress
04.30 hours
CTG (Fig. 4.3)

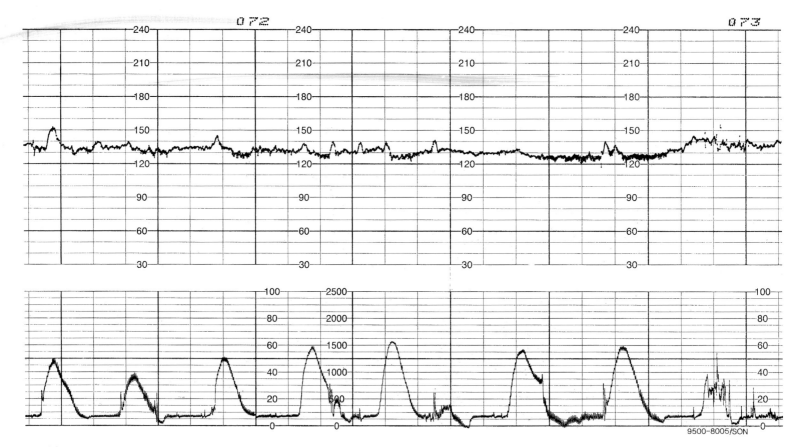

Fig. 4.3

NORMAL

CTG

1 What do you notice about the baseline?
2 What do you notice about the baseline variability?
3 What periodic changes, if any, are present?
4 What do you notice about the uterine activity?
5 What is the most probable cause of fetal heart rate abnormality shown on this trace?
6 What treatment and/or intervention would you consider necessary for this fetal heart rate pattern?

NOTES

1

2

3

4

5

6

ANALYSIS

1 Baseline 130–135 b.p.m.
2 Variability around 5 beats
3 No decelerations, accelerations present
4 Contracting 3–4 in 10 minutes
5 Normal CTG
6 No action necessary

OUTCOME

Progressed to second stage of labour
09.58 hours
Normal delivery
Live boy
Apgar score 9/1 9/5
Birthweight 3.58 kg

4

HISTORY

29-year-old gravida 2, para I

Past history

Nil relevant

Antenatal period

Twin pregnancy diagnosed on booking scan
Admitted at 36 weeks with contractions

Labour

03.10 hours
Cervical os 4 cm dilated
Artificial rupture of membranes — clear liquor
draining
Fetal scalp electrode applied to twin I (faint
line on CTG)
Twin II externally monitored (darker line on
CTG)
Contractions monitored externally
03.50 hours
Epidural analgesia commenced
08.30 hours
Cervical os 8 cm dilated
CTG (Fig. 4.4)

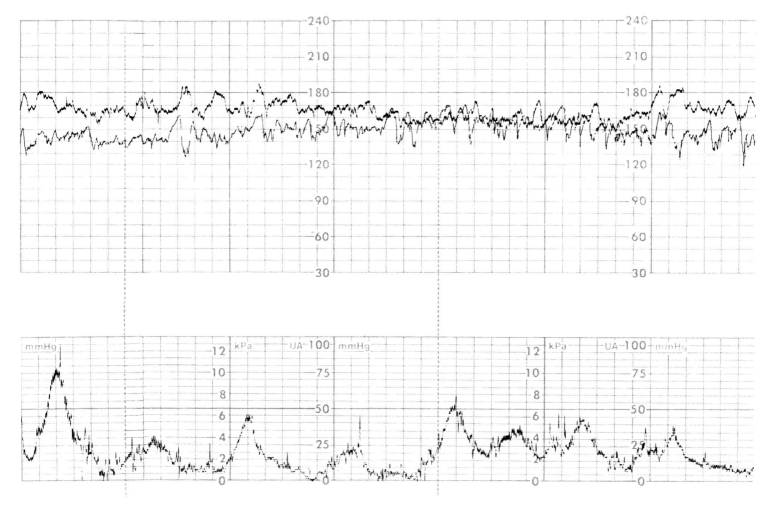

Fig. 4.4

CTG

1 What do you notice about the baseline?
2 What do you notice about the baseline variability?
3 What periodic changes, if any, are present?
4 What do you notice about the uterine activity?
5 What is the most probable cause of fetal heart rate abnormality shown on this trace?
6 What treatment and/or intervention would you consider necessary for this fetal heart rate pattern?

NOTES

1

2

3

4

5

6

1 Baseline
   Twin I: 145–150 b.p.m.
   Twin II: 155–165 b.p.m.
2 Variability
   Twin I: 5–10 b.p.m.
   Twin II: external, therefore not accurate;
   appears 5–10 beats.
3 No decelerations, accelerations present
4 Contracting 3–4 in 10 minutes
5 Normal CTG of both twins
6 No action necessary

09.50 hours
Second stage of labour diagnosed
11.30 hours
Spontaneous vertex delivery of twin I
Live boy
Apgar score 9/1 9/5
Birthweight 2.500 kg
12.20 hours
Straight forceps delivery of twin II
Live boy
Apgar score 9/1 9/5
Birthweight 2.580 kg

5

HISTORY

24-year-old Gravida 4 para 1 + 2

Past History

Previous normal delivery.
Deep vein thrombosis 6 years ago, on Fragmin
(dalteparin sodium)

Antenatal period

Normal
Admitted at 39 weeks gestation in spontaneous
labour

Labour

Vaginal assessment on admission revealed
cervix to be thin and well applied to presenting
part, cervical os was 5 cm dilated.
Membranes intact.
Fetal heart monitored by external transducer.
No analgesia.
CTG (Fig. 4.5)

080695 080696 080697

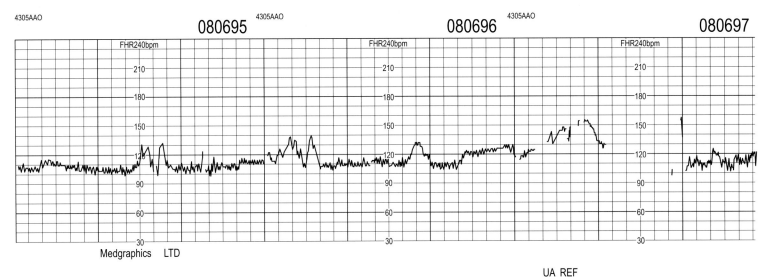

Medgraphics   LTD

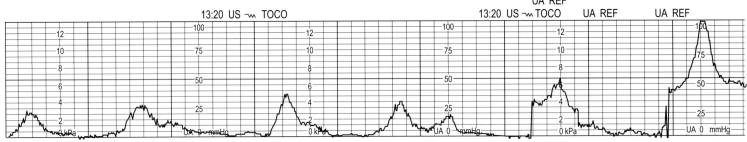

Fig. 4.5

NORMAL

CTG

1 What do you notice about the baseline?
2 What do you notice about the baseline variability?
3 What periodic changes, if any, are present?
4 What do you notice about the uterine activity?
5 What is the most probable cause of fetal heart rate abnormality shown on this trace?
6 What treatment and/or intervention would you consider necessary for this fetal heart rate pattern?

NOTES

1

2

3

4

5

6

NORMAL

1 Baseline 110 b.p.m.
2 Variability 5 to 10 beats
3 None, accelerations with contractions
4 Contracting 1:3
5 Labour

This woman has been deemed as low risk during labour. The reason for continuous fetal heart rate monitoring in labour should be questioned. Following discussion between the woman and her midwife, highlighting best practice guidelines, intermittent auscultation should be offered as the preferred method of fetal heart rate monitoring. If the woman chooses continuous monitoring there must be documentary evidence in the case notes of the risks and benefits that were discussed and that informed consent was gained.

At the end of the portion of CTG, the woman was feeling urges to push. A repeat vaginal assessment revealed the cervix to be thin and well applied to the presenting part. The cervical os was 9 cm dilated. Membranes were ruptured artificially with clear liquor evident.
The CTG remained in progress.
Second stage of labour was diagnosed 15 minutes later. Progress was slow resulting in a straight forceps delivery 2 hours into the second stage.
Live girl, Apgar score 8 and 8

Cord gases	pH	Base excess
UA	7.13	5.5
UV	7.27	6.5

Birthweight 3.260 kg

Bradycardia

HISTORY

24-year-old gravida 2, para I

Past history
Nil relevant

Antenatal period
Normal
Admitted at 41 weeks with contractions for
2 hours

Labour
05.20 hours
Cervical os 2 cm dilated
Fetal scalp electrode applied
Intrauterine pressure catheter inserted
05.40 hours
Epidural analgesia commenced
08.45 hours
Cervical os 6 cm dilated
CTG (Fig. 4.6)

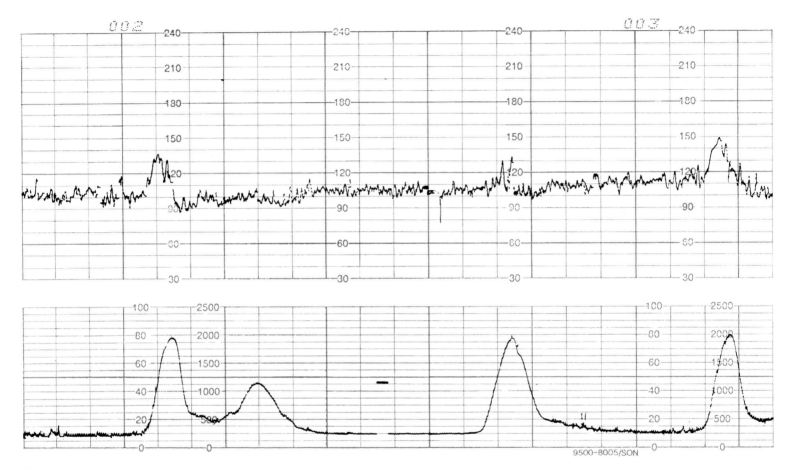

Fig. 4.6

CTG

1 What do you notice about the baseline?
2 What do you notice about the baseline variability?
3 What periodic changes, if any, are present?
4 What do you notice about the uterine activity?
5 What is the most probable cause of fetal heart rate abnormality shown on this trace?
6 What treatment and/or intervention would you consider necessary for this fetal heart rate pattern?

NOTES

1

2

3

4

5

6

ANALYSIS

1 Baseline 100–110 b.p.m.
2 Variability 5–15 b.p.m.
3 No decelerations, some accelerations
4 Contracting 2 in 10 minutes, varying in strength
5 Low baseline, normal variability and accelerations — normal CTG
6 No action necessary
  Observe for further abnormalities

OUTCOME

14.00 hours
Progressed to second stage of labour
16.30 hours
Straight forceps delivery for delay in second stage
Live girl
Apgar score 10/1 10/5
Birthweight 4.250 kg

HISTORY

23-year-old gravida I, para 0

Past history

Nil relevant

Antenatal period

Normal
Admitted at 41 weeks with contractions

Labour

07.00 hours
Cervical os 3 cm dilated
Artificial rupture of membranes — clear liquor draining
Fetal scalp electrode applied
Contractions monitored externally
08.15 hours
CTG (Fig. 4.7)

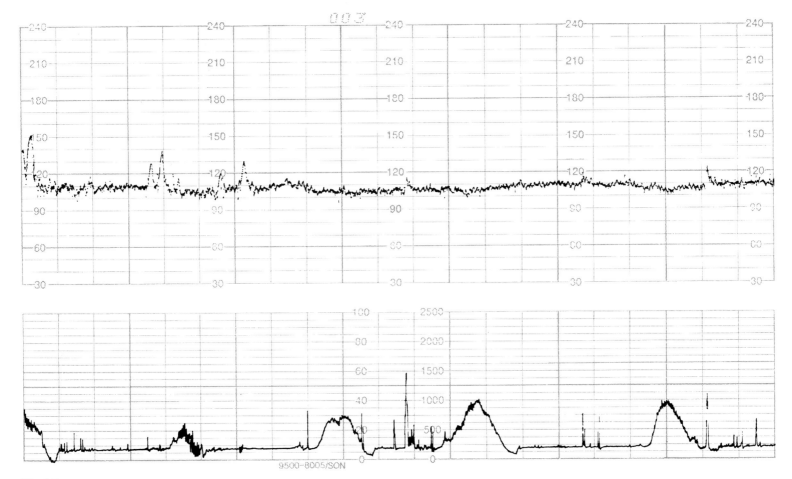

Fig. 4.7

CTG

1 What do you notice about the baseline?
2 What do you notice about the baseline variability?
3 What periodic changes, if any, are present?
4 What do you notice about the uterine activity?
5 What is the most probable cause of fetal heart rate abnormality shown on this trace?
6 What treatment and/or intervention would you consider necessary for this fetal heart rate pattern?

NOTES

1

2

3

4

5

6

BRADYCARDIA

1. Baseline 100–110 b.p.m.
2. Variability less than 5 b.p.m.
3. No decelerations, some accelerations
4. Contracting 2 in 10 minutes, varying in strength
5. Low baseline, variability reduced, although some accelerations are occurring. Normal CTG
6. If variability does not return to within normal limits, fetal blood sampling should be considered

10.00 hours
Cervical os 5 cm dilated
CTG unchanged
Fetal blood sampling attempted — failed
Decision made to deliver
Caesarean section performed
Live boy
Apgar score 9/1 9/5
Birthweight 3.650 kg

HISTORY

27-year-old gravida 4, para 0 + 3

Past history
Three spontaneous mid-trimester abortions

Antenatal period
16 weeks
Cervical cerclage
37 weeks
Cervical suture removed
Admitted at 38 weeks with contractions, since
14.00 hours

Labour
15.00 hours
Cervical os 9.5 cm dilated
Artificial rupture of membranes — clear liquor
draining
Fetal scalp electrode applied
Contractions not monitored
CTG (Fig. 4.8)

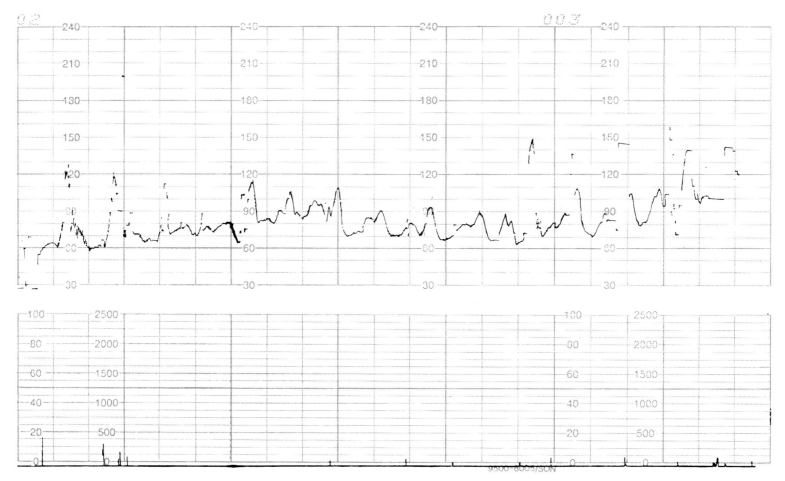

Fig. 4.8

CTG

1 What do you notice about the baseline?
2 What do you notice about the baseline variability?
3 What periodic changes, if any, are present?
4 What do you notice about the uterine activity?
5 What is the most probable cause of fetal heart rate abnormality shown on this trace?
6 What treatment and/or intervention would you consider necessary for this fetal heart rate pattern?

NOTES

1

2

3

4

5

6

ANALYSIS

1 Baseline — difficult to ascertain whether true baseline or prolonged deceleration as no previous CTG
2 Variability little or absent
3 Prolonged deceleration, possible accelerations evident
4 No contractions monitored
5 Rapid progress in labour
   Possible cord compression
6 Change maternal position
   Give facial oxygen
   Exclude cord prolapse
   Prepare for delivery

OUTCOME

15.40 hours
Second stage of labour confirmed
15.50 hours
Straight forceps delivery
Live boy
Apgar score 3/1 9/5
Birthweight 3.200 kg
Cord around neck × 1

Tachycardia

CASE STUDY

9

HISTORY

25-year-old gravida I, para 0

Past history

Nil relevant

Antenatal period

Normal
Admitted at 40 weeks, contracting 1 in
5 minutes for 2 hours

Labour

19.30 hours
Cervical os 3 cm dilated
Artificial rupture of membranes — clear liquor
draining
Fetal scalp electrode applied
Contractions monitored externally
22.30 hours
Cervical os 5 cm dilated
22.45 hours
Epidural analgesia commenced
02.30 hours
Cervical os 6 cm dilated
CTG reactive, baseline 140 b.p.m.
05.30 hours
Cervical os 8 cm dilated
08.30 hours
Cervical os 9.5 cm dilated
Clear liquor draining
Maternal temperature 37.2°C
09.45 hours
Second stage of labour diagnosed
CTG (Fig. 4.9)

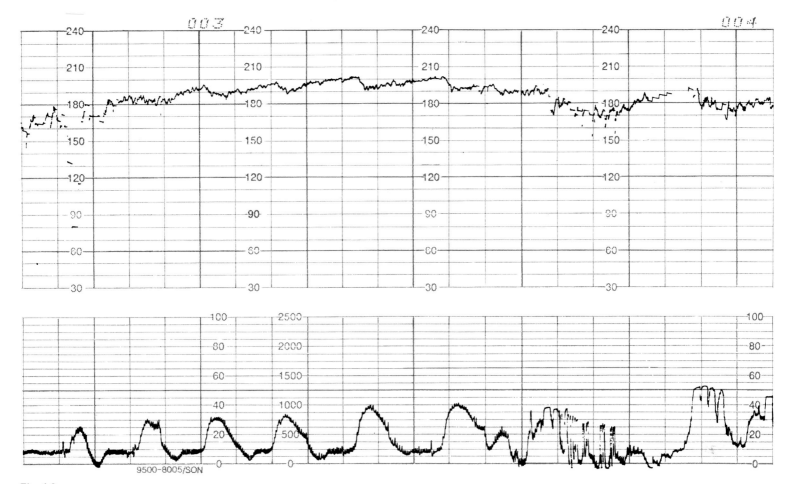

9500-8005/SON

Fig. 4.9

CTG

1 What do you notice about the baseline?
2 What do you notice about the baseline variability?
3 What periodic changes, if any, are present?
4 What do you notice about the uterine activity?
5 What is the most probable cause of fetal heart rate abnormality shown on this trace?
6 What treatment and/or intervention would you consider necessary for this fetal heart rate pattern?

NOTES

1

2

3

4

5

6

ANALYSIS

1 Baseline 190–200 b.p.m.
2 Variability less than 5 b.p.m.
3 No decelerations
4 Contracting 4 in 10 minutes, varying in strength
5 Maternal pyrexia could be responsible for fetal tachycardia
   Diminished variability — fetal hypoxia could be indicated
6 Change maternal position
   Reassess maternal temperature
   If pyrexia is evident, infection must be considered and appropriate treatment initiated
   Fetal blood sampling is contraindicated in view of maternal pyrexia
   Delivery should be expedited

OUTCOME

10.00 hours
Commenced pushing
CTG unchanged
10.30 hours
No progress
Straight forceps delivery
Live girl
Apgar score 7/1 9/5
Birthweight 3.460 kg

HISTORY

34-year-old gravida III, para 0 + 1

Past history

Two previous first trimester abortions
Antenatal period
Normal progress
Admitted at 42 weeks' gestation for surgical induction of labour

Labour

11.00 hours
Artificial rupture of membranes — clear liquor draining
Syntocinon (oxytocin) infusion commenced
Fetal heart and contractions monitored externally
16.00 hours
Cervical os 4 cm dilated
Clear liquor draining
CTG normal, baseline 140 b.p.m.
17.30 hours
Epidural analgesia commenced
19.00 hours
Cervical os 8 cm dilated
CTG normal
21.00 hours
Second stage of labour diagnosed
Maternal temperature 37.6°C, pulse 100 b.p.m.
CTG (Fig. 4.10)

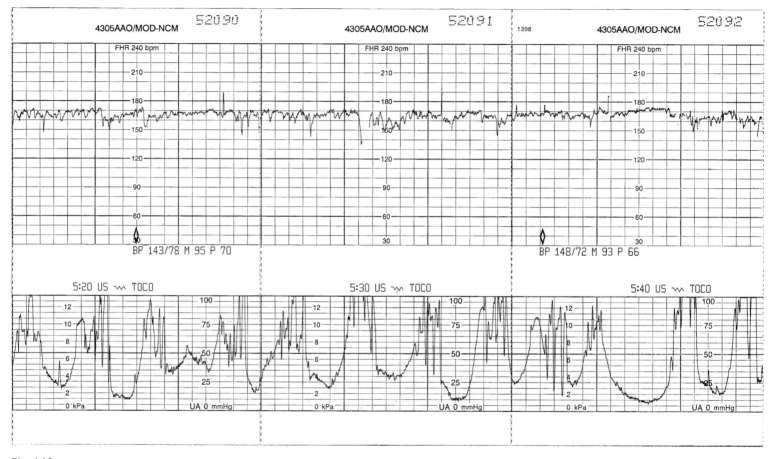

Fig. 4.10

TACHYCARDIA

CTG

1 What do you notice about the baseline?
2 What do you notice about the baseline variability?
3 What periodic changes, if any, are present?
4 What do you notice about the uterine activity?
5 What is the most probable cause of fetal heart rate abnormality shown on this trace?
6 What treatment and/or intervention would you consider necessary for this fetal heart rate pattern?

NOTES

1

2

3

4

5

6

ANALYSIS

1 Baseline 165–170 b.p.m.
2 Variability 5–10, no accelerations
3 No decelerations
4 Contracting 3–4 in 10 minutes
5 Maternal pyrexia
6 Monitor mother's temperature and pulse, record on CTG
  Consider taking blood cultures and treat with antibiotics

OUTCOME

21.30 hours
Commenced pushing
22.15 hours
No progress being made, prepared for instrumental delivery
22.40 hours
Straight forceps delivery
Live boy
Apgar score 5/1 9/5
Birthweight 3.50 kg
Cord gases: pH 7.33, base excess –10.7
Baby's temperature 37.2°C; ear, nose and cord swabs obtained, no growth

HISTORY

36 year old Gravida 2 para 1

Past history
Previous normal delivery

Antenatal period
Normal
Admitted at 40 weeks gestation with
contractions 1:5 for 3 hours.
Vaginal assessment revealed the cervix to be
1 cm long and posterior. The cervical os was
1 cm dilated
CTG (Fig. 4.11)

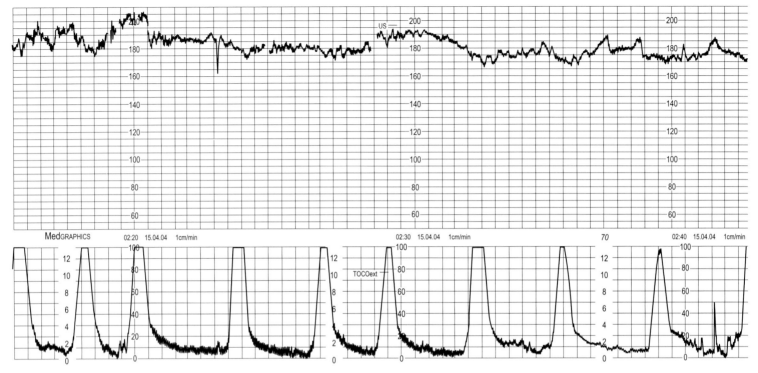

MedGRAPHICS   02:20 15.04.04   1cm/min

US —

TOCOext

70   02:40 15.04.04   1cm/min

02:30 15.04.04   1cm/min

Fig. 4.11

CTG

1 What do you notice about the baseline?
2 What do you notice about the baseline variability?
3 What periodic changes, if any, are present?
4 What do you notice about the uterine activity?
5 What is the most probable cause of fetal heart rate abnormality shown on this trace?
6 What treatment and/or intervention would you consider necessary for this fetal heart rate pattern?

NOTES

1

2

3

4

5

6

1 Baseline 170 to 180 bpm
2 Variability 5 to 10 beats
3 No decelerations, accelerations present
4 Contractions 1:3
5 Maternal pyrexia a possibility. Chronic fetal hypoxia, although all other parameters are within normal limits, so unlikely. Fetal movements are not marked, reactivity to excessive fetal movements cannot be ruled out.
6 Assess maternal temperature and pulse rate.
   Assess fetal movements
   Repeat CTG after 1 hour

Maternal temperature 38.7°C, pulse rate 110 b.p.m.
Paracetomol prescribed regularly
Blood cultures taken and intravenous antibiotics commenced
Pyrexia subsided and fetal tachycardia resolved
Prostin induction of labour was performed the following day
Normal delivery of a live boy occurred 42 hours after admission
Apgar scores 9 and 9
No evidence of infection or chorioamnionitis
Birthweight 4.100 kg

Reduced variability

12

HISTORY

25-year-old gravida I, para 0

Past history
Nil relevant

Antenatal period
Normal
Admitted at 40 weeks with contractions

Labour
19.30 hours
Cervical os 3 cm dilated
Artificial rupture of membranes — clear liquor draining
Fetal scalp electrode applied
Contractions monitored externally
CTG reactive
20.20 hours
Pethidine 100 mg and Sparine 25 mg given intramuscularly
20.40 hours
CTG (Fig. 4.12)

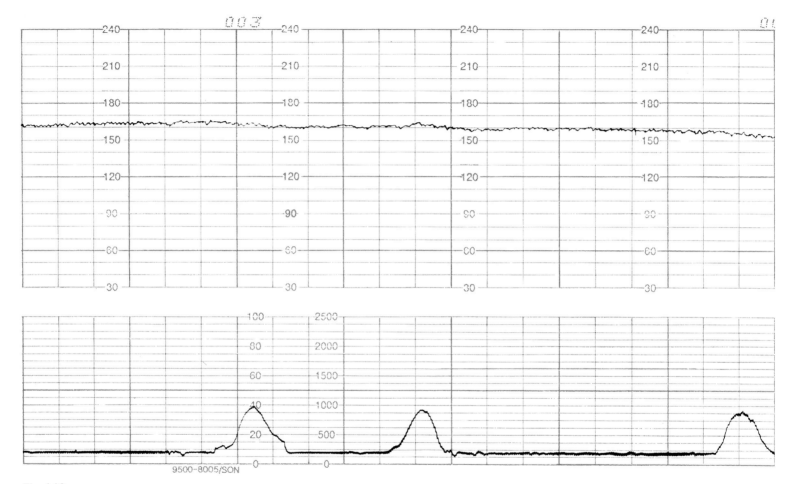

9500-8005/SON

Fig. 4.12

REDUCED VARIABILITY

CTG

1 What do you notice about the baseline?
2 What do you notice about the baseline variability?
3 What periodic changes, if any, are present?
4 What do you notice about the uterine activity?
5 What is the most probable cause of fetal heart rate abnormality shown on this trace?
6 What treatment and/or intervention would you consider necessary for this fetal heart rate pattern?

NOTES

1

2

3

4

5

6

ANALYSIS

1 Baseline 160 b.p.m.
2 Variability little or none present
3 None
4 Contractions irregular, 1–2 in 10 minutes
5 In view of reactive CTG prior to analgesia, probably pethidine induced
6 Observe for further abnormalities If pattern persists for longer than 40 minutes, fetal blood sampling is indicated

OUTCOME

02.00 hours
Cervical os 6 cm dilated
CTG now reactive
07.30 hours
Second stage of labour diagnosed
08.20 hours
Spontaneous vertex delivery
Live girl
Apgar score 7/1 9/5
Birthweight 4.040 kg

CASE STUDY

13

HISTORY

26-year-old gravida 2, para 1

Past history
Nil relevant

Antenatal period
Normal
Admitted at 40 weeks, contracting 1 in 5 minutes

Labour
05.30 hours
Cervical os 1 cm dilated
Admission CTG normal
Allowed to mobilise
09.30 hours
Cervix thick, cervical os 2 cm dilated
Requesting epidural analgesia
Artificial rupture of membranes — clear liquor draining
Fetal scalp electrode applied
Contractions monitored externally
10.25 hours
Epidural analgesia commenced
Occasional mild variable decelerations noted on CTG
13.10 hours
Cervical os 3.5 cm dilated
Liquor clear
CTG (Fig. 4.13)

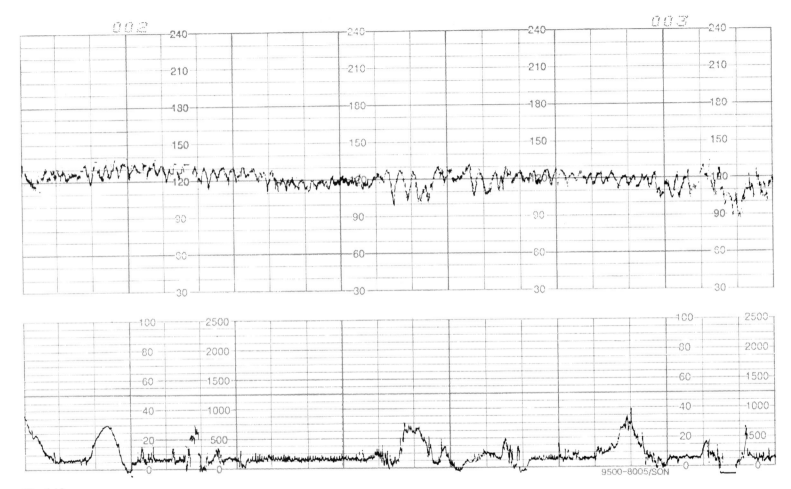

Fig. 4.13

CTG

1 What do you notice about the baseline?
2 What do you notice about the baseline variability?
3 What periodic changes, if any, are present?
4 What do you notice about the uterine activity?
5 What is the most probable cause of fetal heart rate abnormality shown on this trace?
6 What treatment and/or intervention would you consider necessary for this fetal heart rate pattern?

NOTES

1

2

3

4

5

6

ANALYSIS

1 Baseline 125–135 b.p.m.
2 Variability virtually absent; sinusoidal pattern
3 None
4 Contractions irregular, not monitored adequately
5 Preceding variable decelerations — cord occlusion probable, resulting in fetal hypoxia
6 Change maternal posture
  Give facial oxygen
  Increase intravenous fluids
  Fetal blood sampling is indicated
  Prepare for delivery

OUTCOME

14.00 hours
Variable decelerations occur again
Sinusoidal pattern remains
14.25 hours
Fetal blood sampling performed: pH 7.23, base excess –14.3
15.12 hours
Emergency caesarean section performed
Live boy
Apgar score 5/1 9/5
Birthweight 3.620 kg
Umbilical cord wrapped around body

14

HISTORY

32-year-old gravida 4, para 2 + 1

Past history
Previous mid-trimester abortion

Antenatal period
Normal progress
Admitted in spontaneous labour at 39 weeks' gestation

Labour
17.00 hours
Cervical os 5 cm dilated, membranes intact
17.58 hours
Pethidine 100 mg and Sparine 25 mg given intramuscularly
18.00 hours
CTG (Fig. 4.14)

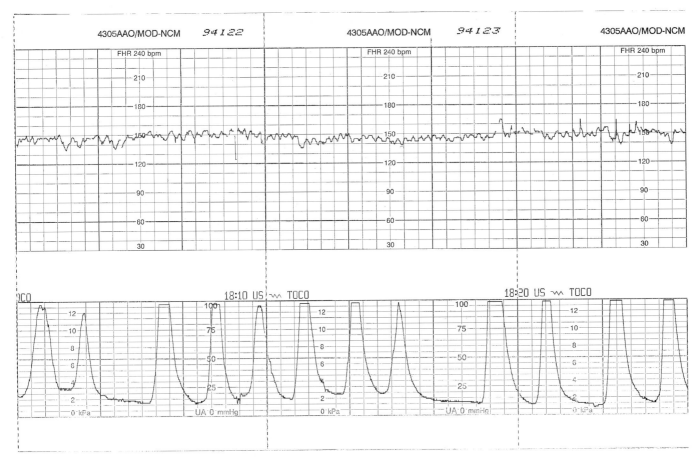

Fig. 4.14

CTG

1 What do you notice about the baseline?
2 What do you notice about the baseline variability?
3 What periodic changes, if any, are present?
4 What do you notice about the uterine activity?
5 What is the most probable cause of fetal heart rate abnormality shown on this trace?
6 What treatment and/or intervention would you consider necessary for this fetal heart rate pattern?

NOTES

1

2

3

4

5

6

ANALYSIS

1 Baseline 145–150 b.p.m.
2 Variability —? sinusoidal pattern initially, reverts to normal variability towards end of portion of CTG with small accelerations
3 No decelerations, possibly small accelerations present
4 Contracting 4 in 10 minutes
5 In view of normal variability previously, return to normal at end of CTG and absence of other abnormalities, probably pethidine induced
6 Continue to monitor the fetal heart
   If pattern persists, consider artificial rupture of the membranes to assess the colour of the liquor

OUTCOME

Progressed rapidly to normal delivery at
19.00 hours
Live boy
Apgar score 9/1 9/5
Birthweight 2.96 kg

15

HISTORY

25-year-old gravida 2, para 0 + 1

Past history
Deep venous thrombosis 4 years ago

Antenatal history
Treated with prophylactic subcutaneous heparin from 16 weeks
Admitted at 40 weeks, contracting 1 in 5 minutes

Labour
16.45 hours
Cervical os 2–3 cm dilated
Artificial rupture of membranes — fresh, thick meconium-stained liquor draining
Fetal scalp electrode applied
Contractions monitored externally
CTG (Fig. 4.15)

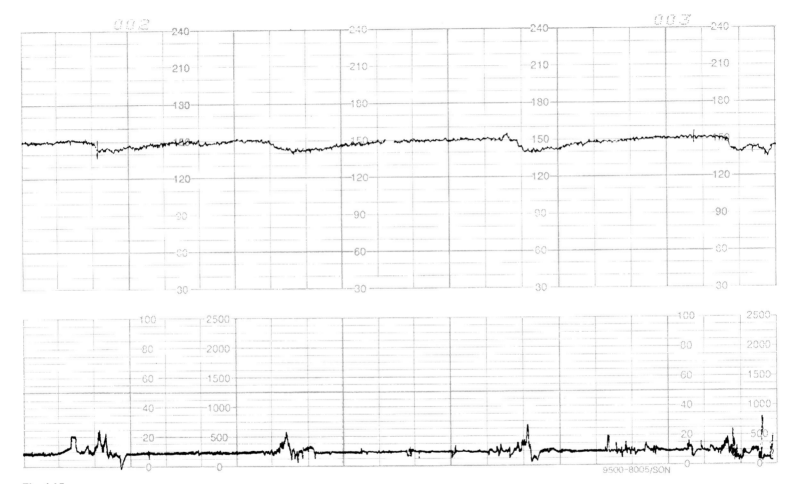

Fig. 4.15

REDUCED VARIABILITY

CTG

1 What do you notice about the baseline?
2 What do you notice about the baseline variability?
3 What periodic changes, if any, are present?
4 What do you notice about the uterine activity?
5 What is the most probable cause of fetal heart rate abnormality shown on this trace?
6 What treatment and/or intervention would you consider necessary for this fetal heart rate pattern?

NOTES

1

2

3

4

5

6

ANALYSIS

1 Baseline 145–150 b.p.m.
2 Variability little or absent
3 Shallow decelerations, cannot be classified as contractions as not monitored adequately
4 Contractions not monitored adequately
5 Decreased variability, decelerations, presence of fresh meconium — fetal hypoxia
6 Change maternal position
  Give facial oxygen
  Prepare for delivery

OUTCOME

17.30 hours
Caesarean section performed
Live boy
Apgar score 8/1 10/5
Birthweight 3.100 kg

16

HISTORY

26-year-old Gravida 2 para 1

Past history

Previous forceps delivery for delay in second stage of labour.
No medical problems

Antenatal period

Normal. Admitted at 37 weeks gestation with a history of diminished fetal movements
over the past 2 days
No signs of labour onset
CTG (Fig. 4.16)

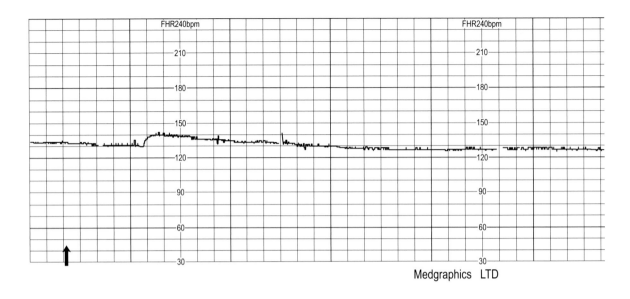

FHR240bpm　　　　　　　　　FHR240bpm

Medgraphics　LTD

S TOCO　　　　　　　　　08:20 US TOCO

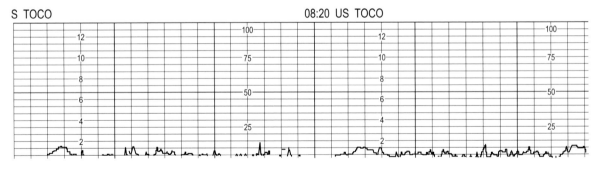

Fig. 4.16

CTG

1 What do you notice about the baseline?
2 What do you notice about the baseline variability?
3 What periodic changes, if any, are present?
4 What do you notice about the uterine activity?
5 What is the most probable cause of fetal heart rate abnormality shown on this trace?
6 What treatment and/or intervention would you consider necessary for this fetal heart rate pattern?

NOTES

1

2

3

4

5

6

1 Baseline 130 b.p.m.
2 Variability absent
3 No decelerations, no accelerations
4 No contractions.
5 The reduced variability could be due to fetal sleep, or sedative drugs. The woman should be asked about any alcohol or drug consumption. However in view of the absent variability and history of altered fetal movements, fetal hypoxia must be considered
6 Continue CTG, if no improvement consider delivery

Maternal observations of blood pressure, pulse and temperature were normal. Vaginal assessment revealed the cervix to be 0.5 cm long, softening and posterior. The cervical os was 2 cm dilated. There was sufficient concern regarding the CTG in this instance that immediate delivery by caesarean section was performed.

A live girl was delivered with an apgar score of 1 and 2.

Cord gases	pH	Base excess
UA	7.28	6.6
UV	7.31	2.3

Birthweight 2.760 kg
This baby sadly died at 3 hours of age.

HISTORY

19-year-old gravida I, para 0

Past history

Nil of note

Antenatal period

Three admissions in mid trimester with low abdominal pain, no cause was found
Admitted at 40 weeks and 3 days gestation with contractions
Vaginal assessment revealed the cervix to be effaced, thin and 4 cm dilated. She was transferred to delivery suite

Labour

Analgesia was requested and pethidine 100 mg was given
35 minutes later CTG, fetal heart rate monitored by external transducer
CTG (Fig. 4.17)

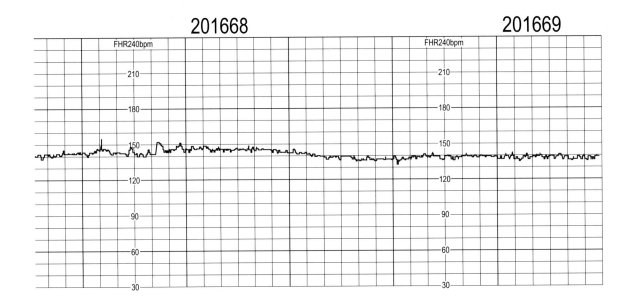

201668   201669

FHR240bpm   FHR240bpm

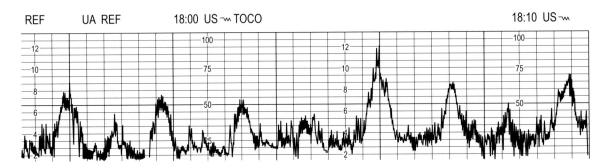

REF   UA REF   18:00 US TOCO   18:10 US

Fig. 4.17

CTG

1 What do you notice about the baseline?
2 What do you notice about the baseline variability?
3 What periodic changes, if any, are present?
4 What do you notice about the uterine activity?
5 What is the most probable cause of fetal heart rate abnormality shown on this trace?
6 What treatment and/or intervention would you consider necessary for this fetal heart rate pattern?

NOTES

1

2

3

4

5

6

1 Baseline 140 b.p.m.
2 Variability less than 5 beats
3 No decelerations, no accelerations
4 Contractions not monitored adequately
5 Loss of fetal heart rate variability following administration of pethidine. Fetal hypoxia should be considered if pattern continues beyond 40 minutes
6 Continue to observe CTG until parameters return to normal, then discontinue. As this woman was deemed low risk for labour the reason why a CTG was commenced should be questioned. The administration of pethidine should not be a reason for a CTG as this may lead to other interventions when a decrease in variability inevitably occurs. The woman should be offered intermittent auscultation as the preferred method of fetal heart rate monitoring. If she chooses to have continuous monitoring the risks and benefits as explained to the woman must be documented in the case notes and her informed consent gained

Progressed well in labour
Variability returned to within normal limits
The CTG was discontinued and intermittent auscultation was used for the remainder of the labour
A live boy was delivered 6 hours following the CTG
Apgar score 9 and 9
Birthweight 3.240 kg

Early
decelerations

HISTORY

21-year-old gravida 2, para 0

Past history

Nil relevant

Antenatal period

Normal
Admitted at 42 weeks in spontaneous labour, contracting 1 in 6 minutes
Cervical os 2–3 cm dilated
21.30 hours
Transferred to ward

Labour

08.00 hours
Cervical os 4 cm dilated
Artificial rupture of membranes — clear liquor draining
Fetal scalp electrode applied
Intrauterine pressure catheter inserted
11.00 hours
Cervical os 6 cm dilated
11.50 hours
Epidural analgesia commenced
13.30 hours
Cervical os 9 cm dilated
15.00 hours
CTG (Fig. 4.18)

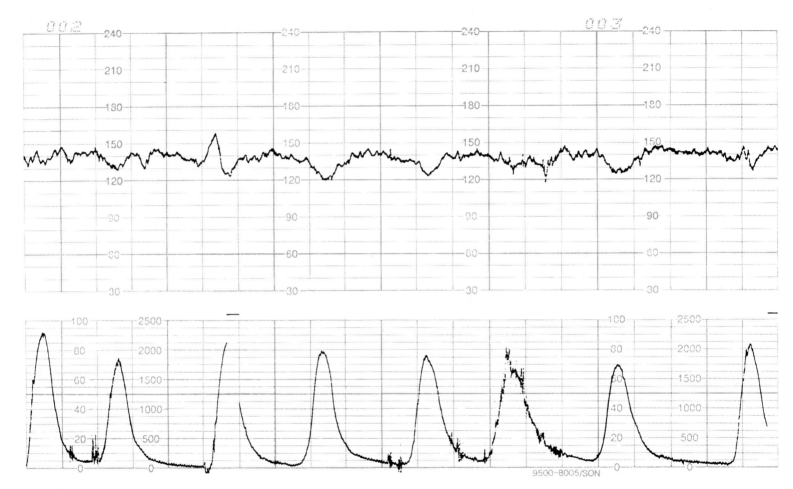

Fig. 4.18

CTG

1 What do you notice about the baseline?
2 What do you notice about the baseline variability?
3 What periodic changes, if any, are present?
4 What do you notice about the uterine activity?
5 What is the most probable cause of fetal heart rate abnormality shown on this trace?
6 What treatment and/or intervention would you consider necessary for this fetal heart rate pattern?

NOTES

1

2

3

4

5

6

ANALYSIS

1 Baseline 140–145 b.p.m.
2 Variability 5 b.p.m.
3 Early decelerations, accelerations present
4 Contracting 4 in 10 minutes, lasting
   90 seconds
5 Head compression
6 Change maternal position
   Observe CTG for further abnormalities

OUTCOME

15.55 hours
Second stage of labour diagnosed
16.55 hours
Commenced pushing
17.45 hours
No progress made
Straight forceps delivery
Live boy
Apgar score 9/1 9/5
Birthweight 4.040 kg

19

HISTORY

24-year-old gravida 2, para 0 + I

Past history
Nil relevant

Antenatal period
Normal
Admitted at 40 weeks
21.00 hours
Spontaneous rupture of membranes — clear liquor draining
Contracting 1 in 5 minutes

Labour
Cervical os 2–3 cm dilated
Fetal scalp electrode applied
Intrauterine pressure catheter inserted
00.15 hours
Cervical os 3 cm dilated
Pethidine 100 mg and Sparine 25 mg given intramuscularly
03.10 hours
Cervical os 5 cm dilated
06.00 hours
Cervical os 7 cm dilated
08.45 hours
Epidural analgesia commenced
09.15 hours
CTG (Fig. 4.19)

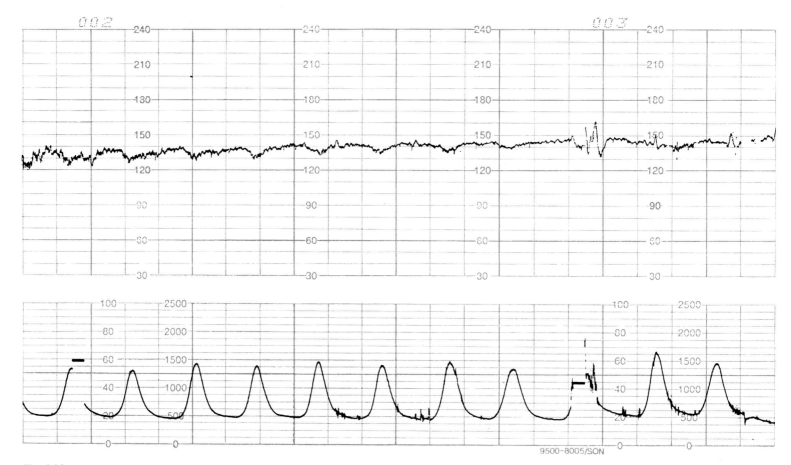

Fig. 4.19

EARLY DECELERATIONS

CTG

1 What do you notice about the baseline?
2 What do you notice about the baseline variability?
3 What periodic changes, if any, are present?
4 What do you notice about the uterine activity?
5 What is the most probable cause of fetal heart rate abnormality shown on this trace?
6 What treatment and/or intervention would you consider necessary for this fetal heart rate pattern?

NOTES

1

2

3

4

5

6

1. Baseline 130–135 b.p.m., rising during CTG
2. Variability less than 5 b.p.m., accelerations with some contractions
3. Shallow early decelerations, one acceleration
4. Contracting 5 in 10 minutes
5. Head compression variability reduced, previously normal, acceleration present — probably sleep phase
6. Change maternal position. If variability does not increase within 40 minutes, fetal blood sampling is indicated

09.45 hours
Second stage of labour diagnosed
Variability now 5–10 b.p.m.
11.00 hours
Commenced pushing
12.02 hours
Spontaneous vertex delivery
Live girl
Apgar score 9/1 9/5
Birthweight 4.220 kg

HISTORY

27-year-old gravida I, para 0

Past history

Nil relevant

Antenatal period

Normal
Admitted at 41 weeks with spontaneous
rupture of membranes — clear liquor draining;
contracting 1 in 5 minutes

Labour

12.45 hours
Cervical os 3 cm dilated
Fetal scalp electrode applied
Intrauterine pressure catheter inserted
14.30 hours
CTG (Fig. 4.20)

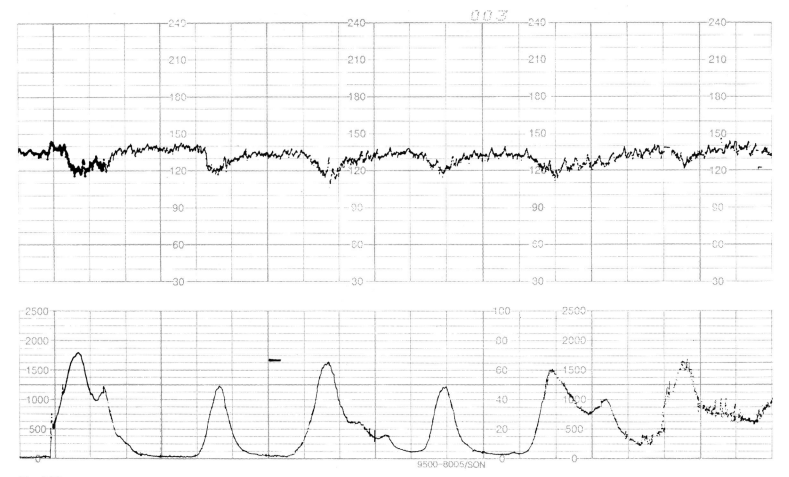

Fig. 4.20

CTG

1 What do you notice about the baseline?
2 What do you notice about the baseline variability?
3 What periodic changes, if any, are present?
4 What do you notice about the uterine activity?
5 What is the most probable cause of fetal heart rate abnormality shown on this trace?
6 What treatment and/or intervention would you consider necessary for this fetal heart rate pattern?

HISTORY

1

2

3

4

5

6

ANALYSIS

1 Baseline 130–135 b.p.m.
2 Variability 5–10 b.p.m.
3 Early decelerations
4 Contracting 1 in 3 minutes, varying in strength
5 Head compression
6 Change maternal position
  Observe for further abnormalities

OUTCOME

15.30 hours
Cervical os 5 cm dilated
16.30 hours
Second stage diagnosed
Commenced pushing
Deep variable decelerations noted
16.55 hours
Rotational forceps delivery
Live girl
Apgar score 6/1 9/5
Birthweight 2.630 kg
Cord around neck × 3

21

HISTORY

27-year-old gravida 3, para 2

Past history
Nil relevant

Antenatal period
Developed mild hypertension in last few weeks of pregnancy. No proteinurea, blood profile normal
Admitted at 41 weeks gestation in spontaneous labour
Vaginal assessment revealed the cervix to be thin, well applied to presenting part and the cervical os 6cm dilated

Labour
Continuous fetal heart rate monitoring was initiated because of the hypertension. The cervical os is now 8 cm dilated
CTG (Fig. 4.21)

073380 073381

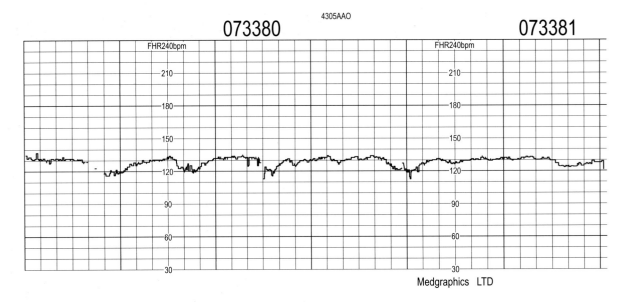

Medgraphics LTD

08:30 US ⌇ TOCO   08:40 US ⌇ TOCO

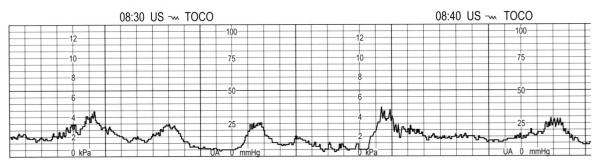

Fig. 4.21

EARLY DECELERATIONS

CTG

1 What do you notice about the baseline?
2 What do you notice about the baseline variability?
3 What periodic changes, if any, are present?
4 What do you notice about the uterine activity?
5 What is the most probable cause of fetal heart rate abnormality shown on this trace?
6 What treatment and/or intervention would you consider necessary for this fetal heart rate pattern?

NOTES

1

2

3

4

5

6

1 Baseline 130–b.p.m.
2 Variability less than 5 beats
3 Early decelerations
4 Contractions 2 to 3 : 10
5 Head compression causing early decelerations. Decreased variability could be due to fetal sleep, if pattern persists beyond 40 minutes, fetal hypoxia should be considered
6 Continue CTG. Change maternal position to relieve head compression. If variability does not improve after 40 minutes consider fetal blood sampling

Variability returned to normal 15 minutes later, with accelerations also present
Labour progresses well and a live girl was born with an apgar score of 9 and 9

Cord gases	pH	Base excess
UA	7.23	4.2
UV	7.35	3.7

Birthweight 3.900 kg

Late decelerations

HISTORY

23-year-old gravida 2, para 1

Past history

Nil relevant

Antenatal period

Normal
Admitted at 39 weeks in spontaneous labour,
contracting 1 in 5 minutes
Admission CTG (Fig. 4.22)

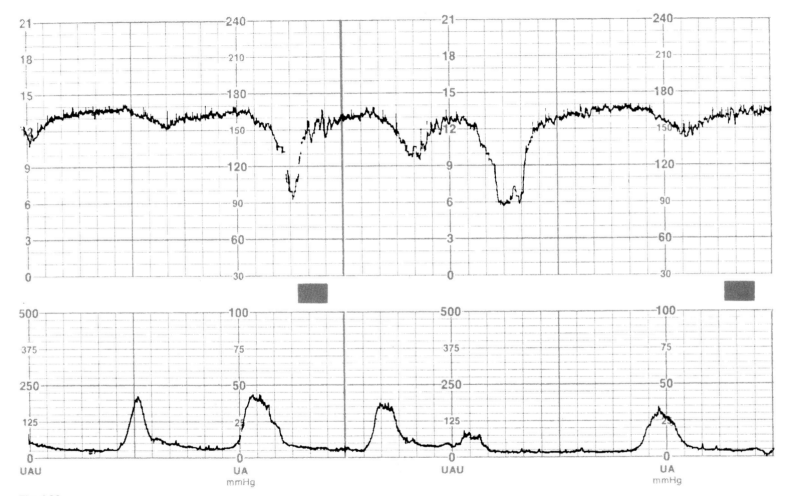

Fig. 4.22

CTG

1 What do you notice about the baseline?
2 What do you notice about the baseline variability?
3 What periodic changes, if any, are present?
4 What do you notice about the uterine activity?
5 What is the most probable cause of fetal heart rate abnormality shown on this trace?
6 What treatment and/or intervention would you consider necessary for this fetal heart rate pattern?

NOTES

1

2

3

4

5

6

1 Baseline 160–165 b.p.m.
2 Variability — external recording, therefore not accurate; appears less than 5 b.p.m.
3 Late decelerations
4 Irregular contractions, 2–3 in 10 minutes
5 Fetal hypoxia
6 Change maternal position
Give facial oxygen
Vaginal examination to assess cervical dilation
Commence intravenous fluids
If cervical os not dilated, consider induction of labour or caesarean section

01.40 hours
Cervical os 5 cm dilated
Artificial rupture of membranes — fresh, thick meconium-stained liquor draining
Fetal scalp electrode applied
CTG — late decelerations continue
02.00 hours
Caesarean section performed
Live boy
Apgar score 2/1 10/5
Birthweight 2.88 kg
Placenta appears unhealthy

HISTORY

27-year-old gravida I, para 0

Past history

Nil relevant

Antenatal period

Normal
Admitted at 41 weeks with history of
diminished fetal movements for 3 days
Mild contractions for 2 hours
Admission CTG (Fig. 4.23)

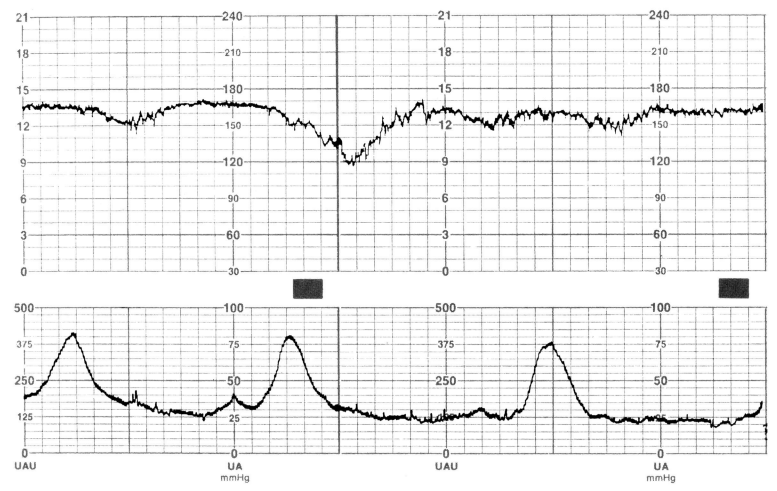

Fig. 4.23

CTG

1 What do you notice about the baseline?
2 What do you notice about the baseline variability?
3 What periodic changes, if any, are present?
4 What do you notice about the uterine activity?
5 What is the most probable cause of fetal heart rate abnormality shown on this trace?
6 What treatment and/or intervention would you consider necessary for this fetal heart rate pattern?

NOTES

1

2

3

4

5

6

ANALYSIS

1 Baseline 160–165 b.p.m.
2 Variability — externally monitored, therefore not accurate; appears reduced
3 Late decelerations
4 Contracting 1–2 in 10 minutes
5 Fetal hypoxia
  Note history of diminished fetal movements
6 Change maternal position
  Give facial oxygen
  Vaginal examination to assess cervical dilation
  If cervix favourable, artificial rupture of membranes to assess the colour of the liquor and to perform fetal blood sampling
  Prepare for delivery while these actions are performed
  If cervix not favourable, deliver

OUTCOME

24.00 hours
Cervical os 5 cm dilated
Artificial rupture of membranes — fresh meconium-stained liquor draining
Fetal scalp electrode applied — resulting CTG of poor quality
Fetal blood sampling performed: pH 7.09, base excess −10
01.48 hours
Caesarean section performed
Live boy
Apgar score 4/1 8/5
Birthweight 3.330 kg

CASE STUDY

24

HISTORY

25-year-old gravida I, para 0

Past history

Nil relevant

Antenatal period

Normal
Admitted in spontaneous labour at 41 weeks, contracting 1 in 5 minutes

Labour

16.30 hours
Cervical os 2 cm dilated
Artificial rupture of membrane — clear liquor draining
Fetal scalp electrode applied
Contractions monitored externally
17.30 hours
CTG (Fig. 4.24)

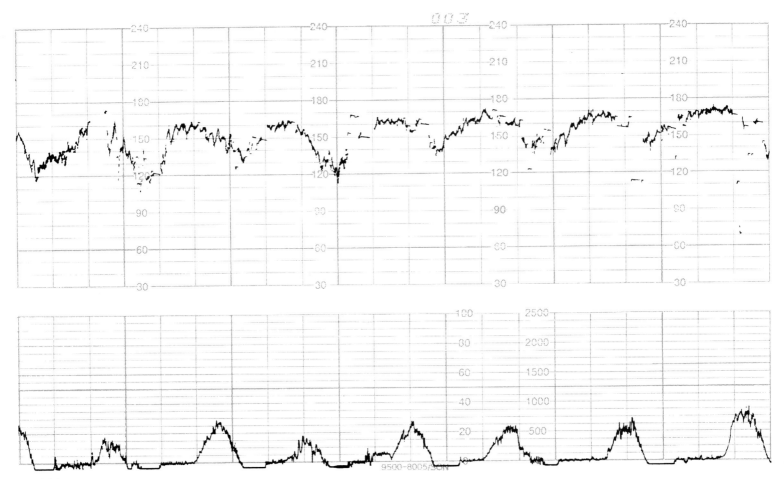

Fig. 4.24

LATE DECELERATIONS

CTG

1 What do you notice about the baseline?
2 What do you notice about the baseline variability?
3 What periodic changes, if any, are present?
4 What do you notice about the uterine activity?
5 What is the most probable cause of fetal heart rate abnormality shown on this trace?
6 What treatment and/or intervention would you consider necessary for this fetal heart rate pattern?

NOTES

1

2

3

4

5

6

1 Baseline 160–165 b.p.m.
2 Variability 5 b.p.m.
3 Late decelerations
4 Contracting 3 in 10 minutes, not
   adequately monitored
5 Fetal hypoxia
6 Change maternal position
   Give facial oxygen
   Commence intravenous infusion
   Fetal blood sampling is indicated
   As baseline tachycardia present with
   decreased variability, prepare for delivery
   while these actions are being performed

18.00 hours
Fetal blood sampling performed: pH 7.32
18.30 hours
Meconium-stained liquor noted
Late decelerations now more prolonged
19.00 hours
Second stage of labour diagnosed
19.15 hours
Rotational forceps delivery
Live boy
Apgar score 8/1 9/5
Birthweight 3.700 kg
Large number of placental infarcts noted

25

HISTORY

37-year-old gravida V, para 3 + 1

Past history

Insulin-dependent, diabetic for 6 years

Antenatal period

Amniocentesis at 17 weeks — indication, maternal age
Two admissions for control of diabetes

Labour

Surgical induction at 38 weeks
10.45 hours
Cervix 1.5 cm long, cervical os 1.5 cm dilated
Artificial rupture of membranes — clear liquor draining
Fetal scalp electrode applied
Intrauterine pressure catheter inserted
Syntocinon (oxytocin) infusion commenced
14.50 hours
Cervical os 4 cm dilated
15.15 hours
Epidural analgesia commenced
16.50 hours
Syntocinon (oxytocin) infusing at 8 mU/min.
Contractions now monitored externally
CTG (Fig. 4.25)

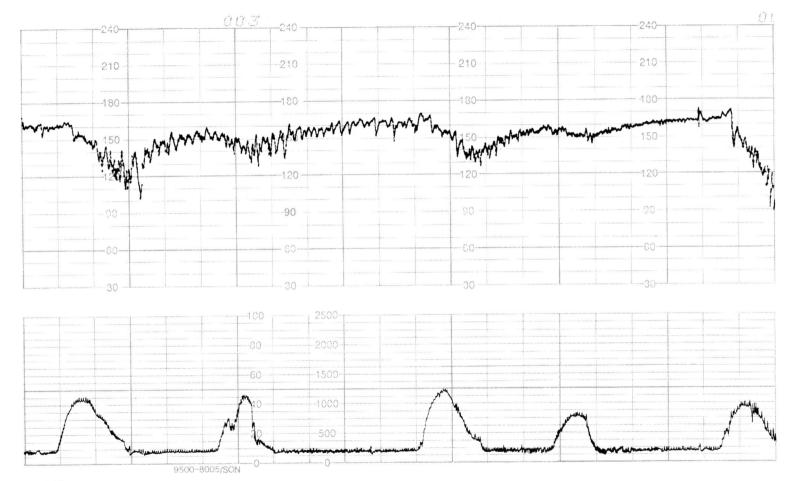

Fig. 4.25

9500-8005/SON

CTG

1 What do you notice about the baseline?
2 What do you notice about the baseline variability?
3 What periodic changes, if any, are present?
4 What do you notice about the uterine activity?
5 What is the most probable cause of fetal heart rate abnormality shown on this trace?
6 What treatment and/or intervention would you consider necessary for this fetal heart rate pattern?

NOTES

1

2

3

4

5

6

ANALYSIS

1 Baseline 150–160 b.p.m.
2 Variability appears reduced, possibly sinusoidal pattern in places
3 Late decelerations
4 Contractions 2–3 in 10 minutes, varying in strength
5 Fetal hypoxia
   Note maternal diabetes
6 Change maternal position
   Give facial oxygen
   Increase intravenous infusion
   Take sample of blood for glucose level
   Fetal blood sampling is indicated
   Prepare for delivery

OUTCOME

17.15 hours
Fetal blood sampling performed: pH 7.28, base excess –6
Blood glucose estimation 4 mmol/L
CTG — pattern continues
17.58 hours
Caesarean section performed
Live boy
Apgar score 9/1 9/5
Birthweight 3.500 kg

Variable decelerations

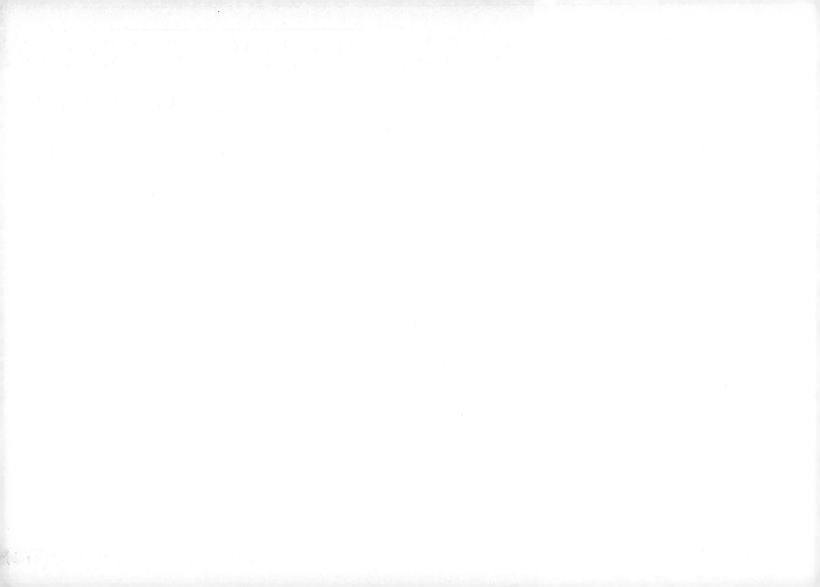

HISTORY

20-year-old gravida I, para 0

Past history

Nil relevant

Antenatal period

Normal
Admitted at 40 weeks with contractions for
3 hours

Labour

05.30 hours
Cervical os 5 cm dilated
Artificial rupture of membranes — clear liquor
draining
Fetal scalp electrode applied
Intrauterine pressure catheter inserted
06.45 hours
Pethidine 100 mg and Sparine 25 mg given
intramuscularly
08.35 hours
Cervical os 6 cm dilated
10.15 hours
Epidural analgesia commenced
11.00 hours
Cervical os 9 cm dilated
12.30 hours
CTG (Fig. 4.26)

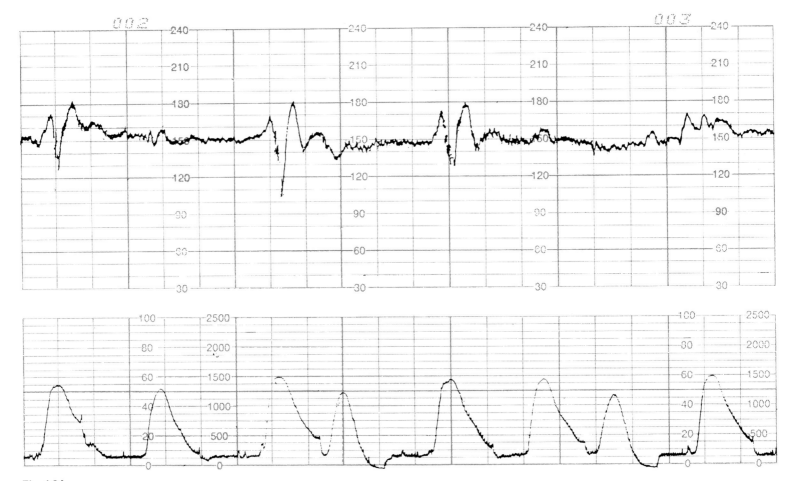

Fig. 4.26

CTG

1 What do you notice about the baseline?
2 What do you notice about the baseline variability?
3 What periodic changes, if any, are present?
4 What do you notice about the uterine activity?
5 What is the most probable cause of fetal heart rate abnormality shown on this trace?
6 What treatment and/or intervention would you consider necessary for this fetal heart rate pattern?

NOTES

1

2

3

4

5

6

ANALYSIS

1 Baseline 145–150 b.p.m.
2 Variability less than 5 b.p.m.
3 Variable decelerations, acceleration precedes and follows deceleration
4 Contracting 4–5 in 10 minutes
5 Cord compression
6 Change maternal position
  Give facial oxygen
  Increase intravenous infusion
  Observe for further abnormalities
  If variability decreases any further, or if decelerations become more severe, fetal blood sampling is indicated

OUTCOME

13.00 hours
Second stage of labour diagnosed
13.30 hours
Commenced pushing
14.25 hours
No progress made
Straight forceps delivery
Live boy
Apgar score 9/1 9/5
Birthweight 3.250 kg
Cord around neck × 1

HISTORY

25-year-old gravida I, para 0

Past history

Nil relevant

Antenatal period

Normal
Admitted at 41 weeks, contracting 1 in
5 minutes

Labour

10.30 hours
Cervical os 7 cm dilated
Artificial rupture of membranes — clear liquor
draining
Fetal scalp electrode applied
12.50 hours
Cervical os 8 cm dilated
Epidural analgesia commenced
14.30 hours
CTG (Fig. 4.27)

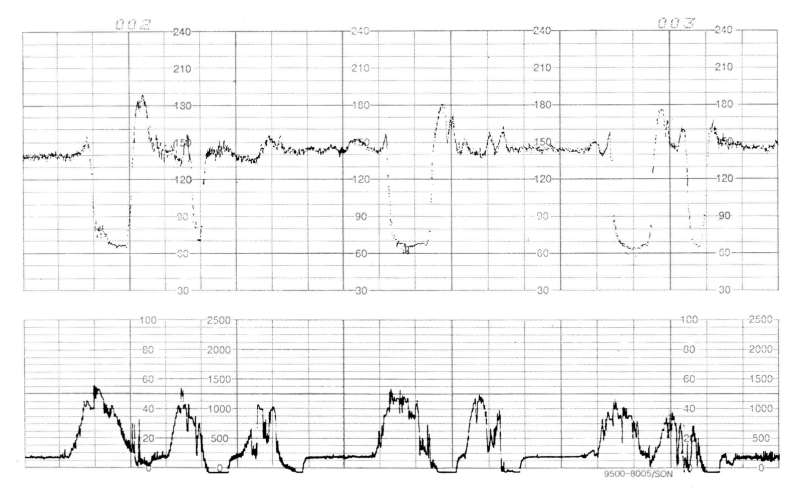

Fig. 4.27

VARIABLE DECELERATIONS

CTG

1 What do you notice about the baseline?
2 What do you notice about the baseline variability?
3 What periodic changes, if any, are present?
4 What do you notice about the uterine activity?
5 What is the most probable cause of fetal heart rate abnormality shown on this trace?
6 What treatment and/or intervention would you consider necessary for this fetal heart rate pattern?

NOTES

1

2

3

4

5

6

1 Baseline 140–145 b.p.m.
2 Variability 5 b.p.m., some accelerations
3 Variable decelerations, accelerations present
4 Contracting 3 in 10 minutes, varying in strength
5 Cord compression
6 Change maternal position
   Give facial oxygen
   Vaginal examination to assess cervical dilation and exclude cord prolapse
   Fetal blood sampling is indicated

14.45 hours
Second stage of labour diagnosed
Fetal blood sampling performed: pH 7.29, base excess −6
15.05 hours
Commenced pushing
15.30 hours
No improvement in CTG
15.42 hours
Straight forceps delivery
Live girl
Apgar score 3/1 8/5
Birthweight 3.060 kg
Cord around neck × 1

HISTORY

28-year-old gravida I, para 0

Past history

Nil relevant

Antenatal period

Normal
Admitted at 41 weeks, contracting 1 in
5 minutes, spontaneous rupture of membranes

Labour

03.30 hours
Cervical os 4 cm dilated
Clear liquor draining
Fetal scalp electrode applied
Contractions monitored externally
04.00 hours
Epidural analgesia commenced
05.30 hours
Second stage diagnosed
06.30 hours
Commenced pushing
07.00 hours
No progress being made
CTG (Fig. 4.28)

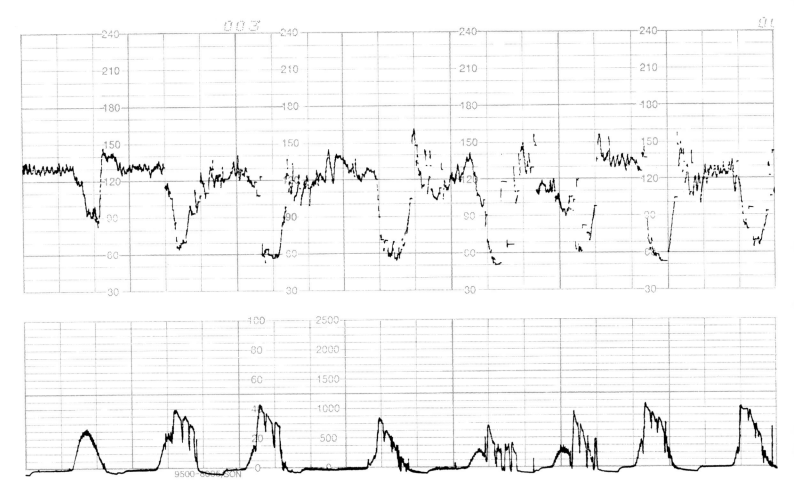

Fig. 4.28

VARIABLE DECELERATIONS

CTG

1 What do you notice about the baseline?
2 What do you notice about the baseline variability?
3 What periodic changes, if any, are present?
4 What do you notice about the uterine activity?
5 What is the most probable cause of fetal heart rate abnormality shown on this trace?
6 What treatment and/or intervention would you consider necessary for this fetal heart rate pattern?

NOTES

1

2

3

4

5

6

ANALYSIS

1 Baseline 125–130 b.p.m.
2 Variability 5–10 b.p.m.
3 Variable decelerations, accelerations present
4 Contracting 3–4 in 10 minutes
5 Cord compression
6 Change maternal position
Give facial oxygen
Increase intravenous infusion
In view of little progress being made, prepare for delivery

OUTCOME

07.40 hours
Straight forceps delivery
Live girl
Apgar score 9/1 9/5
Birthweight 2.840 kg
Cord around neck × 1

HISTORY

27-year-old gravida I, para 0

Past history
Nil relevant

Antenatal period
Subchorionic bleed noted at 29 weeks on ultrasound scan
Follow-up scans normal
Pregnancy progressed well
Admitted at term plus 11 days for surgical induction of labour

Labour
10.00 hours
Artificial rupture of membranes — clear liquor draining
Initial external CTG normal
10.45 hours
Syntocinon (oxytocin) infusion commenced
Continuous external CTG commenced
16.30 hours
Epidural analgesia in progress
CTG normal
01.15 hours
Cervical os 7 cm dilated, clear liquor draining
Progress in labour slow
01.50 hours
CTG (Fig. 4.29)

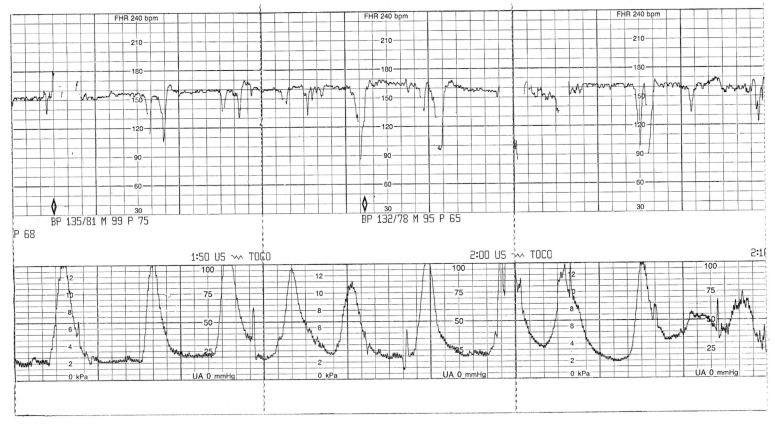

Fig. 4.29

VARIABLE DECELERATIONS

CTG

1 What do you notice about the baseline?
2 What do you notice about the baseline variability?
3 What periodic changes, if any, are present?
4 What do you notice about the uterine activity?
5 What is the most probable cause of fetal heart rate abnormality shown on this trace?
6 What treatment and/or intervention would you consider necessary for this fetal heart rate pattern?

NOTES

1

2

3

4

5

6

1 Baseline 155–160 b.p.m.
2 Variability less than 5, no accelerations
3 Variable decelerations
4 Contracting 3–4 in 10 minutes
5 Cord compression
Baseline slightly raised although has
remained constant throughout labour
6 Change maternal position
Record maternal temperature and pulse
rate
Fetal blood sampling may be indicated if
pattern persists

Mother apyrexial, pulse rate 92 b.p.m.
Variable decelerations reduce, occasional
decelerations only
05.00 hours
Progressed to second stage of labour
06.50 hours
No progress made with maternal effort
Cephalic presentation still one-fifth palpable
abdominally
Occasional variable decelerations continue
Emergency caesarean section performed
Live boy
Apgar score 9/1 9/5
Birthweight 3.840 kg
Cord gases: pH 7.40, base excess −3.2

HISTORY

32-year-old gravida 2, para 2

Past history

Caesarean section 3 years ago for twin
pregnancy

Antenatal period

Normal
Admitted at 42 weeks with spontaneous
rupture of membranes and contractions

Labour

23.55 hours
Cervical os 2 cm dilated — clear liquor
draining
Fetal scalp electrode applied
Contractions monitored externally
00.10 hours
Pethidine 100 mg and Sparine 25 mg given
intramuscularly
02.15 hours
Cervical os 4 cm dilated
Intrauterine pressure catheter inserted
03.00 hours
CTG (Fig. 4.30)

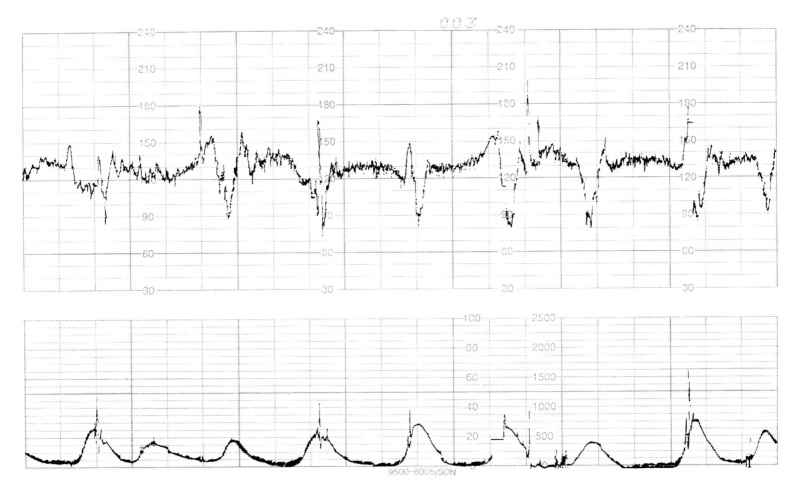

Fig. 4.30

VARIABLE DECELERATIONS

CTG

1 What do you notice about the baseline?
2 What do you notice about the baseline variability?
3 What periodic changes, if any, are present?
4 What do you notice about the uterine activity?
5 What is the most probable cause of fetal heart rate abnormality shown on this trace?
6 What treatment and/or intervention would you consider necessary for this fetal heart rate pattern?

NOTES

1

2

3

4

5

6

1 Baseline 125–135 b.p.m.
2 Variability 5–10 b.p.m.
3 Variable decelerations, accelerations
  present
4 Contracting 4 in 10 minutes
5 Cord compression
6 Change maternal position
  Give facial oxygen
  Increase intravenous infusion
  Observe for further abnormalities
  If pattern persists, fetal blood sampling is
  indicated

04.00 hours
Cervical os 9 cm dilated
Loop of cord in front of head
Transferred to theatre; second stage of labour
diagnosed on arrival
04.17 hours
Straight forceps delivery
Live boy
Apgar score 8/1 9/5
Birthweight 3.380 kg

Prolonged decelerations

HISTORY

33-year-old gravida 2, para I

Past history

Nil relevant

Antenatal period

Normal
Admitted at 36 weeks with abdominal pain,
fresh bleeding per vagina and contracting 1 in
3 minutes
Speculum examination performed – 30 mL of
fresh blood in vagina
Ultrasound scan performed – upper segment
placenta

Labour

04.30 hours
Cervical os 3 cm dilated
Artificial rupture of membranes — heavily
blood-stained liquor
Fetal scalp electrode applied
Intrauterine pressure catheter inserted
04.55 hours
CTG (Fig. 4.31)

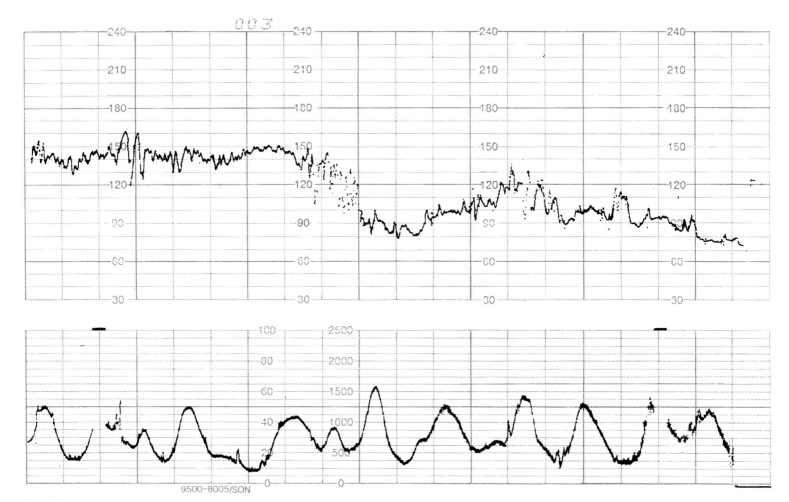

Fig. 4.31

PROLONGED DECELERATIONS

CTG

1 What do you notice about the baseline?
2 What do you notice about the baseline variability?
3 What periodic changes, if any, are present?
4 What do you notice about the uterine activity?
5 What is the most probable cause of fetal heart rate abnormality shown on this trace?
6 What treatment and/or intervention would you consider necessary for this fetal heart rate pattern?

NOTES

1

2

3

4

5

6

ANALYSIS

1 Baseline 135–145 b.p.m.
2 Variability 5–15 b.p.m.
3 Prolonged deceleration
4 Contracting 5 in 10 minutes, varying in strength
5 Possible further placental abruption resulting in diminished oxygen transfer to the fetus, causing fetal hypoxia
6 Vaginal examination to assess cervical dilation
  Change maternal position
  Give facial oxygen
  Prepare for delivery

OUTCOME

05.25 hours
Caesarean section performed
Live boy
Apgar score 3/1 10/5
Birthweight 2.610 kg
300 mL retroplacental clot

HISTORY

23-year-old gravida 2, para 0 + 1

Past history
Nil relevant

Antenatal period
Normal
Admitted at 41 weeks with spontaneous rupture of membranes – slightly meconium-stained liquor draining

Labour
21.40 hours
Cervical os 4 cm dilated
Fetal scalp electrode applied
Contractions monitored externally
22.20 hours
Epidural analgesia commenced
23.15 hours
Cervical os 6 cm dilated
23.30 hours
Epidural top-up given
24.00 hours
Occasional variable decelerations noted
00.50 hours
CTG (Fig. 4.32)

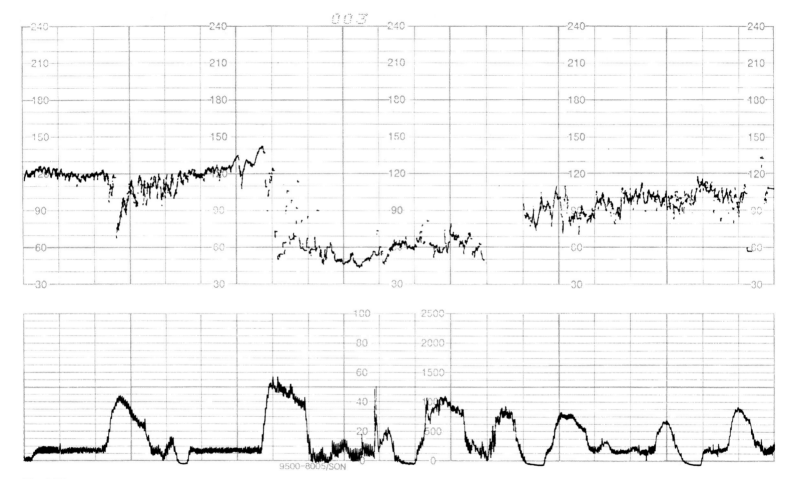

Fig. 4.32

CTG

1 What do you notice about the baseline?
2 What do you notice about the baseline variability?
3 What periodic changes, if any, are present?
4 What do you notice about the uterine activity?
5 What is the most probable cause of fetal heart rate abnormality shown on this trace?
6 What treatment and/or intervention would you consider necessary for this fetal heart rate pattern?

NOTES

1

2

3

4

5

6

ANALYSIS

1 Baseline 120 b.p.m.
2 Variability 5 b.p.m.
3 Prolonged decelerations
4 Contracting 4–5 in 10 minutes, varying in strength
5 Previous variable decelerations — cord occlusion probable, resulting in fetal hypoxia
6 Vaginal examination to assess cervical dilation and to exclude cord prolapse
   Change maternal position
   Give facial oxygen
   Fetal blood sampling when deceleration recovers
   If no recovery, deliver

OUTCOME

Cervical os 8 cm dilated
No cord prolapse
Fetal blood sampling attempted — failed
Fetal heart returned to baseline 120–130 b.p.m., with occasional variable decelerations
03.33 hours
Second stage of labour diagnosed
04.15 hours
Spontaneous vertex delivery
Live boy
Apgar score 1/1 7/5
Birthweight 3.140 kg
True knot in cord

HISTORY

21-year-old gravida I, para 0

Past history

Ovarian cystectomy 3 years ago

Antenatal period

Normal
Admitted at 39 weeks, contracting 1 in
5 minutes for 3 hours

Labour

11.30 hours
Cervical os 2 cm dilated
Artificial rupture of membranes — clear liquor
draining
Fetal scalp electrode applied
Intrauterine pressure catheter inserted
14.30 hours
Cervical os 4 cm dilated
Epidural analgesia commenced
15.30 hours
Epidural top-up given
16.15 hours
CTG (Fig. 4.33)

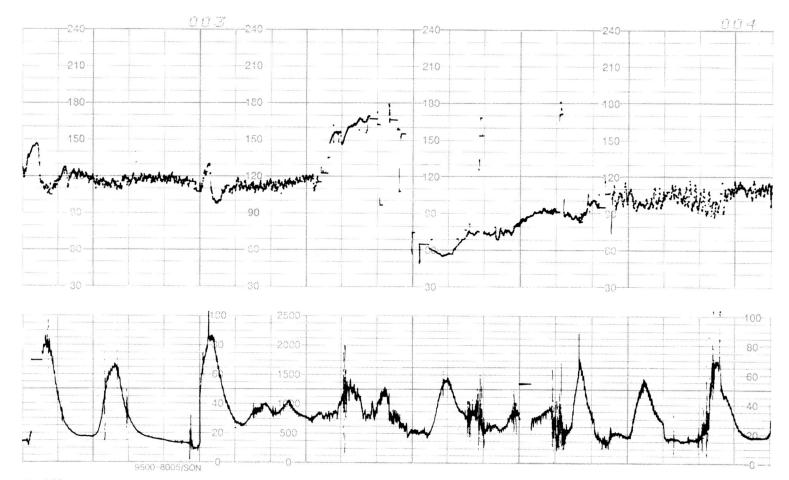

Fig. 4.33

CTG

1 What do you notice about the baseline?
2 What do you notice about the baseline variability?
3 What periodic changes, if any, are present?
4 What do you notice about the uterine activity?
5 What is the most probable cause of fetal heart rate abnormality shown on this trace?
6 What treatment and/or intervention would you consider necessary for this fetal heart rate pattern?

NOTES

1

2

3

4

5

6

ANALYSIS

1 Baseline 110–120 b.p.m.
2 Variability 5–10 b.p.m.
3 Prolonged deceleration, accelerations present prior to this
4 Contracting 4–5 in 10 minutes, varying in strength
5 Deceleration occurs immediately after vaginal examination
6 Change maternal position
  Give facial oxygen
  Increase intravenous fluids
  Consider fetal blood sampling when fetal heart rate returns to normal
  If no recovery, prepare for delivery
  Observe for further abnormalities

OUTCOME

CTG returns to normal — no further decelerations
18.15 hours
Second stage of labour diagnosed
19.40 hours
Straight forceps delivery
Live girl
Apgar score 9/1 9/5
Birthweight 3.480 kg
No cord around neck

Complex

HISTORY

30-year-old gravida I, para 0

Past history

Nil relevant

Antenatal period

Normal
Admitted at 40 weeks with contractions for 2 hours
Early decelerations noted on admission CTG

Labour

22.00 hours
Cervical os 3 cm dilated
Artificial rupture of membranes — clear liquor draining
Fetal scalp electrode applied
Intrauterine pressure catheter inserted
22.30 hours
Epidural analgesia commenced
24.00 hours
Variable decelerations noted
Cervical os 7 cm dilated
01.25 hours
Second stage diagnosed
Commenced pushing
02.00 hours
CTG (Fig. 4.34)

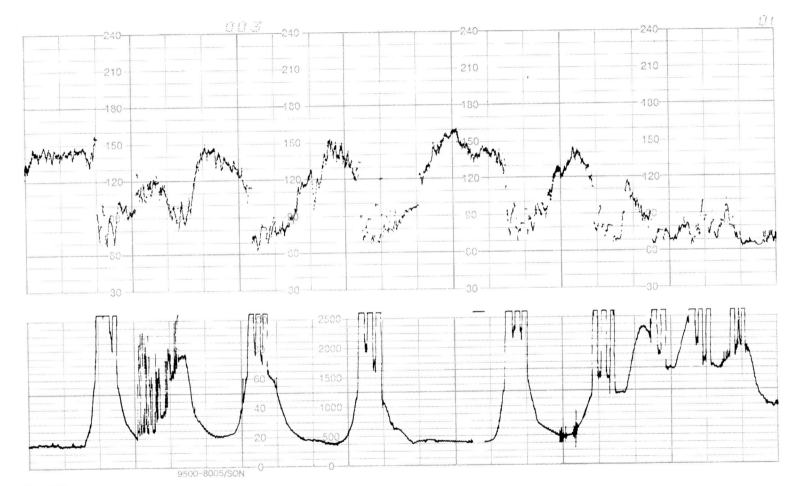

Fig. 4.34

CTG

1 What do you notice about the baseline?
2 What do you notice about the baseline variability?
3 What periodic changes, if any, are present?
4 What do you notice about the uterine activity?
5 What is the most probable cause of fetal heart rate abnormality shown on this trace?
6 What treatment and/or intervention would you consider necessary for this fetal heart rate pattern?

NOTES

1

2

3

4

5

6

ANALYSIS

1 Baseline 145–150 b.p.m.
2 Variability 5–10 b.p.m.
3 Variable decelerations followed by prolonged deceleration
4 Contracting 3–4 in 10 minutes, varying in strength
5 Variable decelerations followed by prolonged deceleration — cord occlusion
6 Change maternal position
  Give facial oxygen
  Increase intravenous fluids
  Prepare for delivery

OUTCOME

02.26 hours
Straight forceps delivery
Live boy
Apgar score 9/1 9/5
Birthweight 3.100 kg
Cord around neck × 2 tightly

CASE STUDY

35

Part 1

HISTORY

19-year-old gravida I, para 0

Past history
Nil relevant

Antenatal period
Normal
Admitted at 40 weeks with spontaneous rupture of membranes and contractions

Labour
09.00 hours
Cervical os 3 cm dilated
Clear liquor draining
Fetal scalp electrode applied
Intrauterine pressure catheter inserted
09.20 hours
Epidural analgesia commenced
13.30 hours
Cervical os 4–5 cm dilated
Variable decelerations noted, baseline
125 b.p.m.
Fetal blood sampling performed: pH 7.32, base excess –2
Syntocinon (oxytocin) infusion commenced
17.00 hours
Cervical os 8 cm dilated
Liquor clear
Maternal temperature 38.8°C
Syntocinon (oxytocin) infusing at 18 mU/min
18.15 hours
CTG (Fig. 4.35 part 1)

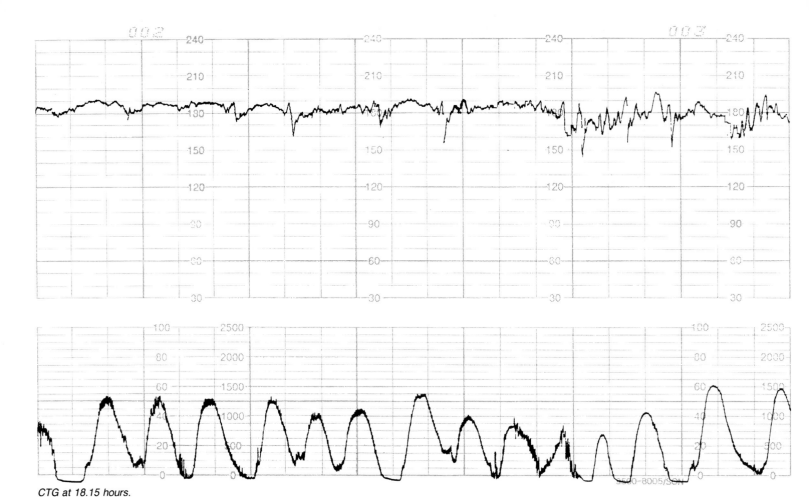

CTG at 18.15 hours.

Fig. 4.35 part I CTG at 18.15 hours.

CTG

1 What do you notice about the baseline?
2 What do you notice about the baseline variability?
3 What periodic changes, if any, are present?
4 What do you notice about the uterine activity?
5 What is the most probable cause of fetal heart rate abnormality shown on this trace?
6 What treatment and/or intervention would you consider necessary for this fetal heart rate pattern?

NOTES

1

2

3

4

5

6

COMPLEX

ANALYSIS

1 Baseline 180–190 b.p.m.
2 Variability 5–10 b.p.m.
3 No decelerations
4 Contracting 8 in 10 minutes
5 Variability normal, no decelerations, uncomplicated tachycardia – maternal pyrexia probable
6 Syntocinon (oxytocin) infusion should be decreased in view of uterine hyperactivity Observe for further abnormalities

OUTCOME

Labour continued
19.00 hours
Cervical os 8 cm dilated
Liquor discoloured:
? pus
? meconium
20.30 hours
Cervical os 8 cm dilated
Cephalic presentation; three-fifths palpable above pelvic brim
Syntocinon (oxytocin) infusing at 10 mU/min
CTG – see Part 2, page 184.

CASE STUDY

35

Part 2

OUTCOME [CONTINUED]

20.30 hours
CTG (Fig. 4.35 part 2)

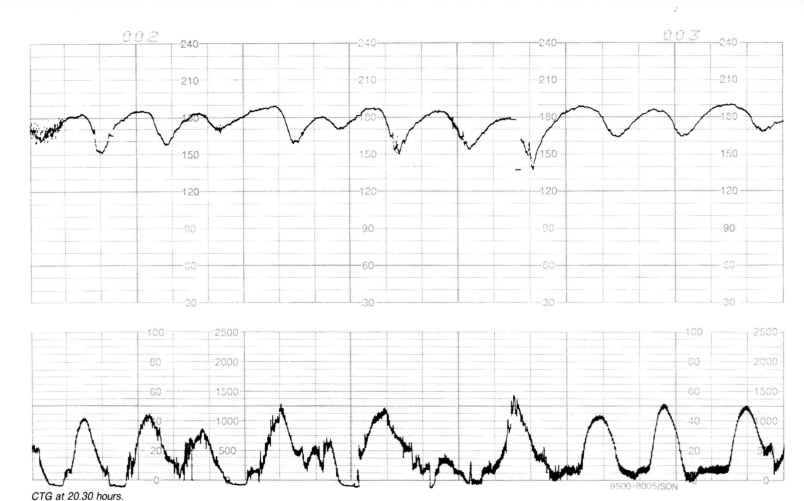

CTG at 20.30 hours.

Fig. 4.35 part 2 CTG at 20.30 hours.

COMPLEX

CTG

1 What do you notice about the baseline?
2 What do you notice about the baseline variability?
3 What periodic changes, if any, are present?
4 What do you notice about the uterine activity?
5 What is the most probable cause of fetal heart rate abnormality shown on this trace?
6 What treatment and/or intervention would you consider necessary for this fetal heart rate pattern?

NOTES

1

2

3

4

5

6

ANALYSIS

1. Baseline 180–190 b.p.m.
2. Variability virtually absent
3. Late decelerations
4. Contracting 4 in 10 minutes
5. Fetal tachycardia, late decelerations, loss of variability — fetal hypoxia
6. Change maternal position
   Give facial oxygen
   Increase intravenous fluids
   Prepare for delivery

OUTCOME

21.55 hours
Caesarean section performed
Live boy
Apgar score 1/1 9/5
Birthweight 4.200 kg
Cord around neck × 2, tightly
Fresh, thick meconium noted at delivery
Placenta appears very gritty and unhealthy

HISTORY

29-year-old gravida I, para 0

Past history
Nil relevant

Antenatal period
Admitted at 39 weeks, history of diminished fetal movements for 3 days
Admission CTG (Fig. 4.36)

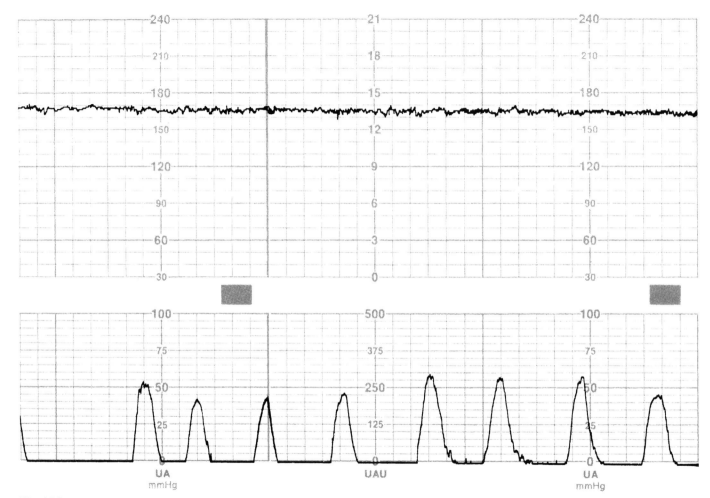

Fig. 4.36

CTG

1 What do you notice about the baseline?
2 What do you notice about the baseline variability?
3 What periodic changes, if any, are present?
4 What do you notice about the uterine activity?
5 What is the most probable cause of fetal heart rate abnormality shown on this trace?
6 What treatment and/or intervention would you consider necessary for this fetal heart rate pattern?

NOTES

1

2

3

4

5

6

1 Baseline 165 b.p.m.
2 Variability — external recording, therefore not accurate; appears virtually absent
3 None
4 Tightening 4–5 in 10 minutes, not painful
5 In view of history of diminished fetal movements, fetal hypoxia probable
6 Change maternal position
  Give facial oxygen
  Vaginal examination to assess cervical dilation, with a view to performing artificial rupture of membranes to observe colour of the liquor
  Prepare for delivery

Cervix posterior, 1 cm long, os 0.5 cm dilated
Caesarean section performed
Live girl
Apgar score 1/1 5/5
Birthweight 2.980 kg
Thick, fresh meconium noted at delivery
Baby transferred to neonatal unit
Listeriosis diagnosed at 2 days old; subsequently recovered

HISTORY

28-year-old gravida I, para 0

Past history

Nil relevant

Antenatal period

Mild hypertension from 36 weeks
No proteinurea
Prostin induction of labour at 39 weeks'
gestation

Labour

04.00 hours
Cervical os 4 cm dilated
Artificial rupture of membranes performed —
clear liquor draining
Epidural analgesia commenced
Continuous external fetal monitoring in
progress
05.10 hours
CTG (Fig. 4.37)

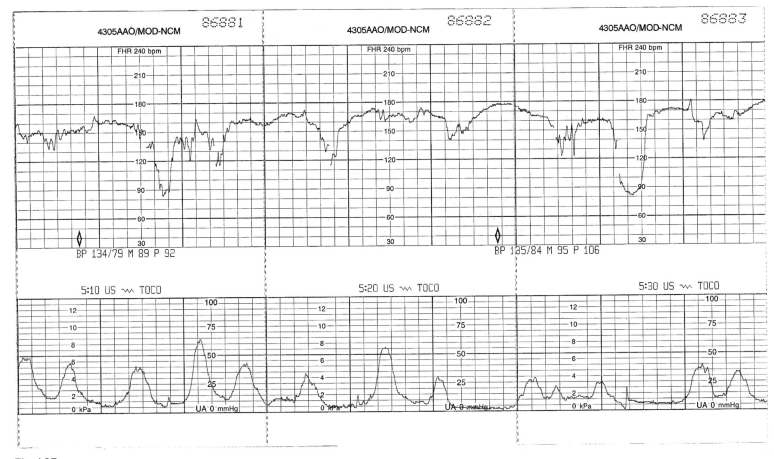

Fig. 4.37

CTG

1 What do you notice about the baseline?
2 What do you notice about the baseline variability?
3 What periodic changes, if any, are present?
4 What do you notice about the uterine activity?
5 What is the most probable cause of fetal heart rate abnormality shown on this trace?
6 What treatment and/or intervention would you consider necessary for this fetal heart rate pattern?

NOTES

1

2

3

4

5

6

1 Baseline initially 160 b.p.m. rising to 180 b.p.m.
2 Variability less than 5, no accelerations
3 Variable decelerations
4 Contracting 3–4 in 10 minutes, irregular in strength and frequency
5 Cord compression
   Fetal tachycardia may be due to maternal pyrexia, although in view of increasing baseline and reduction in variability, fetal hypoxia should be excluded
6 Record maternal temperature
   Change maternal position
   Administer facial oxygen
   Discontinue any oxytocic infusion
   Consider fetal blood sampling

Maternal temperature 37.5°C
Variable decelerations persist, with tachycardia, variability improves
06.10 hours
Fetal blood sampling performed: pH 7.34, base excess –3.6
09.00 hours
Cervical os 8–9 cm dilated
09.30 hours
Maternal temperature now 36.8°C
CTG as before
Repeat fetal blood sampling performed:
pH 7.37, base excess –3.1
10.15 hours
Cervical os 8 cm dilated, therefore decision made for emergency caesarean section
Live girl
Apgar score 7/1 9/5
Birthweight 3.320 kg
Cord gases: pH 7.34, base excess –2.7

HISTORY

26-year-old gravida 2, para 0 + 1

Past history

Nil relevant

Antenatal period

Normal
Admitted at 41 weeks for surgical induction of labour

Labour

12.30 hours
Cervix 0.5 cm long, cervical os 2 cm dilated
Artificial rupture of membranes — clear liquor draining
Fetal scalp electrode applied
Intrauterine pressure catheter inserted
13.45 hours
Epidural analgesia commenced
15.00 hours
Cervix unchanged from 12.30 hours
Syntocinon (oxytocin) infusion commenced
17.00 hours
Cervical os 3–4 cm dilated
19.15 hours
Cervical os 9 cm dilated
21.15 hours
Cervical os 9 cm dilated
Syntocinon (oxytocin) infusing at 8 mU/min
CTG (Fig. 4.38)

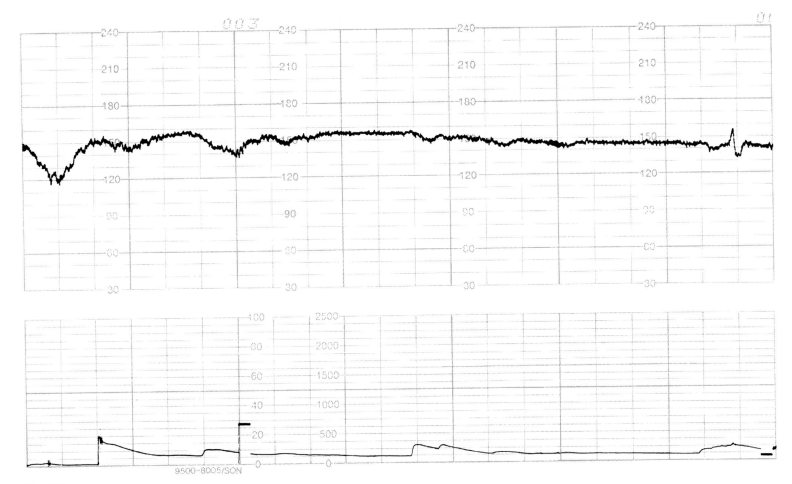

Fig. 4.38

9500-8005/SON

CTG

1 What do you notice about the baseline?
2 What do you notice about the baseline variability?
3 What periodic changes, if any, are present?
4 What do you notice about the uterine activity?
5 What is the most probable cause of fetal heart rate abnormality shown on this trace?
6 What treatment and/or intervention would you consider necessary for this fetal heart rate pattern?

NOTES

1

2

3

4

5

6

ANALYSIS

1 Baseline 140–145 b.p.m.
2 Variability less than 5 b.p.m.
3 Some decelerations initially, cannot be classified as no contractions monitored
4 Contractions not monitored adequately
5 CTG normal to this point
   Decreased variability could be due to fetal sleep; cause for decelerations cannot be identified until they are classified
6 Change maternal position
   Give facial oxygen
   If pattern continues for 40 minutes or longer, fetal blood sampling is indicated

OUTCOME

00.30 hours
Second stage of labour diagnosed
Umbilical cord in vagina
Transferred to theatre
Rotational forceps delivery attempted — failed
Caesarean section performed
Live boy
Apgar score 9/1 9/5
Birthweight 4.100 kg

HISTORY

20-year-old gravida I, para 0

Past history

Nil relevant

Antenatal period

Breech presentation confirmed on ultrasound scan at 38 weeks
Admitted in labour at 39 weeks, contracting 1 in 5 minutes

Labour

23.30 hours
Cervical os 4 cm dilated
Artificial rupture of membranes — clear liquor draining
Fetal scalp electrode applied
Intrauterine pressure catheter inserted
00.57 hours
Epidural analgesia commenced
02.00 hours
Cervical os 7 cm dilated
CTG reactive
Baseline 150 b.p.m.
03.00 hours
Meconium-stained liquor noted
Maternal temperature 36°C
03.50 hours
Cervical os 9.5 cm dilated
CTG (Fig. 4.39)

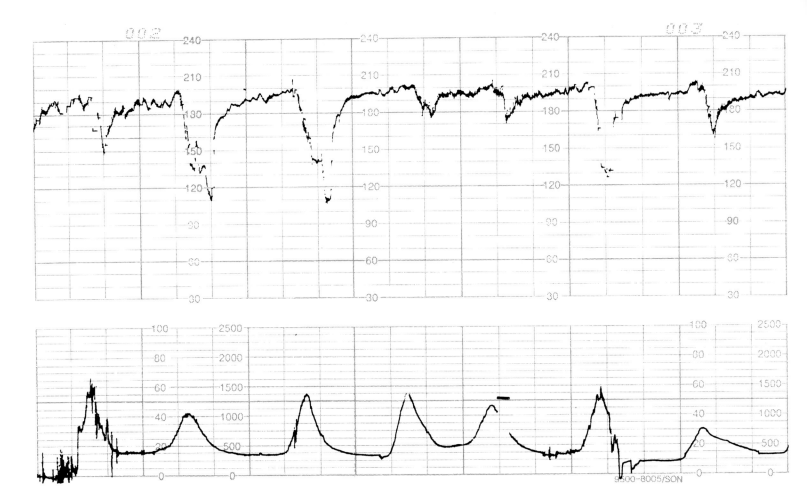

Fig. 4.39

CTG

1 What do you notice about the baseline?
2 What do you notice about the baseline variability?
3 What periodic changes, if any, are present?
4 What do you notice about the uterine activity?
5 What is the most probable cause of fetal heart rate abnormality shown on this trace?
6 What treatment and/or intervention would you consider necessary for this fetal heart rate pattern?

NOTES

1

2

3

4

5

6

ANALYSIS

1 Baseline 190–200 b.p.m.
2 Variability 5 b.p.m.
3 Variable decelerations
4 Contracting 4 in 10 minutes
5 Maternal temperature normal. Baseline increasing, variability diminishing, variable decelerations — fetal hypoxia should be considered
6 Prepare for delivery
  Change maternal position
  Give facial oxygen
  Increase intravenous fluids

OUTCOME

04.30 hours
Caesarean section performed
Live boy
Apgar score 6/1 9/5
Birthweight 3.430 kg

HISTORY

16-year-old gravida I, para 0

Past history
Nil relevant

Antenatal period
Normal
Admitted at 41 weeks with contractions for 5 hours

Labour
17.05 hours
Cervical os 4 cm dilated
Artificial rupture of membranes — clear liquor draining
Fetal scalp electrode applied
Intrauterine pressure catheter inserted
17.15 hours
Pethidine 100 mg and Sparine 25 mg given intramuscularly
19.15 hours
Cervical os 4 cm dilated
Syntocinon (oxytocin) infusion commenced
22.00 hours
Cervical os 4 cm dilated
24.00 hours
Cervical os 4 cm dilated
Clear liquor
Syntocinon infusing at 8 mU/min
Maternal temperature 36.4°C
CTG (Fig. 4.40)

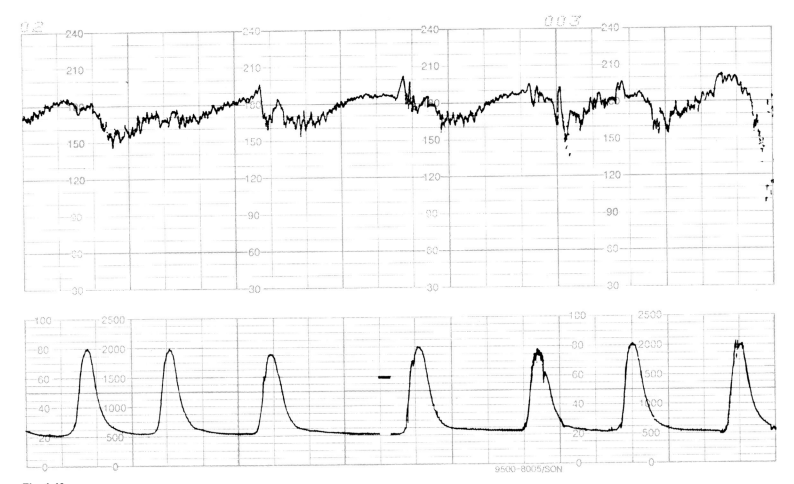

Fig. 4.40

CTG

1 What do you notice about the baseline?
2 What do you notice about the baseline variability?
3 What periodic changes, if any, are present?
4 What do you notice about the uterine activity?
5 What is the most probable cause of fetal heart rate abnormality shown on this trace?
6 What treatment and/or intervention would you consider necessary for this fetal heart rate pattern?

NOTES

1

2

3

4

5

6

ANALYSIS

1 Baseline 180–190 b.p.m.
2 Variability 5–10 b.p.m.
3 Late decelerations, some accelerations
4 Contracting 3–4 in 10 minutes
5 Fetal tachycardia, maternal temperature normal, late decelerations — fetal hypoxia despite variability being within normal limits
6 Change maternal position
 Give facial oxygen
 Increase intravenous infusion
 Stop Syntocinon (oxytocin) infusion
 Fetal blood sampling is indicated
 Prepare for delivery, particularly in view of failure to progress

OUTCOME

02.00 hours
Cervix 6 cm dilated
Fetal blood sampling performed: pH 7.23, base excess –6
CTG continues as before, late decelerations becoming more severe
03.00 hours
Caesarean section performed
Live girl
Apgar score 7/1 10/5
Birthweight 3.240 kg

CASE STUDY

41

HISTORY

18-year-old gravida I, para 0

Past history

Nil relevant

Antenatal period

Normal

Admitted at 36 weeks with history of heavy, fresh bleeding per vagina for 2 hours — sudden onset; complaining of abdominal pain

On examination: abdomen tense and tender; moderate amount fresh bleeding per vagina

Admission CTG (Fig. 4.41)

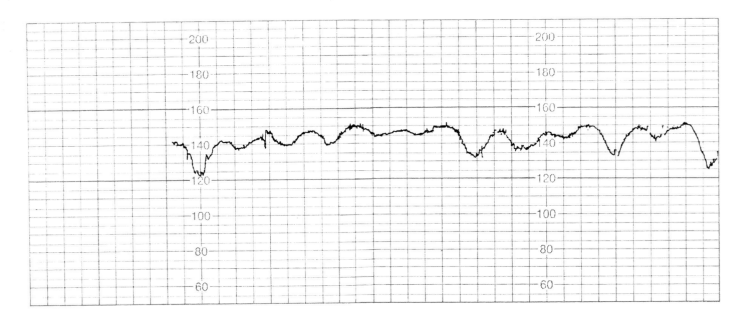

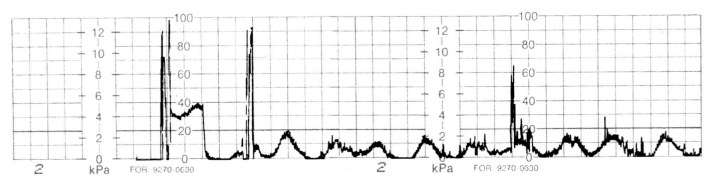

Fig. 4.41

CTG

1 What do you notice about the baseline?
2 What do you notice about the baseline variability?
3 What periodic changes, if any, are present?
4 What do you notice about the uterine activity?
5 What is the most probable cause of fetal heart rate abnormality shown on this trace?
6 What treatment and/or intervention would you consider necessary for this fetal heart rate pattern?

NOTES

1

2

3

4

5

6

1 Baseline 145–150 b.p.m.
2 Variability — external recording, therefore not accurate; appears to be little or absent
3 Late decelerations
4 Uterine irritability
5 Reduced placental blood flow due to placental abruption – fetal hypoxia
6 Prepare for delivery
   Change maternal position
   Give facial oxygen

Ultrasound scan performed — posterior upper segment of placenta
Cervix 1 cm long, cervical os 2 cm dilated
Caesarean section performed
Baby girl
Apgar score 0/1 7/5 9/10
Resuscitated successfully
Birthweight 2.690 kg
Couvelaire uterus noted
Baby discharged at 3 weeks

CASE STUDY

42

HISTORY

36-year-old gravida 3, para 2

Past history

Nil relevant

Antenatal period

Admitted at 33 weeks with raised blood pressure
Diminished fetal movements
Ultrasound scan shows asymmetrical growth retardation and reduced liquor volume
Admission CTG (Fig. 4.42)

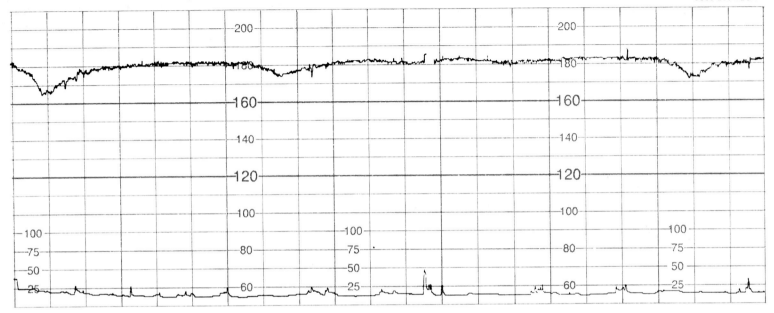

Fig. 4.42

COMPLEX

CTG

1 What do you notice about the baseline?
2 What do you notice about the baseline variability?
3 What periodic changes, if any, are present?
4 What do you notice about the uterine activity?
5 What is the most probable cause of fetal heart rate abnormality shown on this trace?
6 What treatment and/or intervention would you consider necessary for this fetal heart rate pattern?

NOTES

1

2

3

4

5

6

1 Baseline 180 b.p.m.
2 Variability — external recording, therefore not accurate; appears to be virtually absent
3 Shallow decelerations, cannot be classified in absence of contractions
4 No contractions
5 History of intrauterine growth retardation, diminished liquor volume, diminished fetal movements, fetal tachycardia, decreased variability, decelerations occurring without contractions — fetal hypoxia
6 Give facial oxygen
Change maternal position
Prepare for delivery

Emergency caesarean section performed
Live boy
Apgar score 1/1 4/5
Birthweight 1.470 kg
True knot in cord
Baby transferred to neonatal unit
Discharged at 4 weeks

CASE STUDY

43

Part 1

HISTORY

27-year-old gravida 2, para 1

Past history

Nil relevant

Antenatal period

Normal
Admitted at 43 weeks for routine CTG
(Fig. 4.43 part 1)

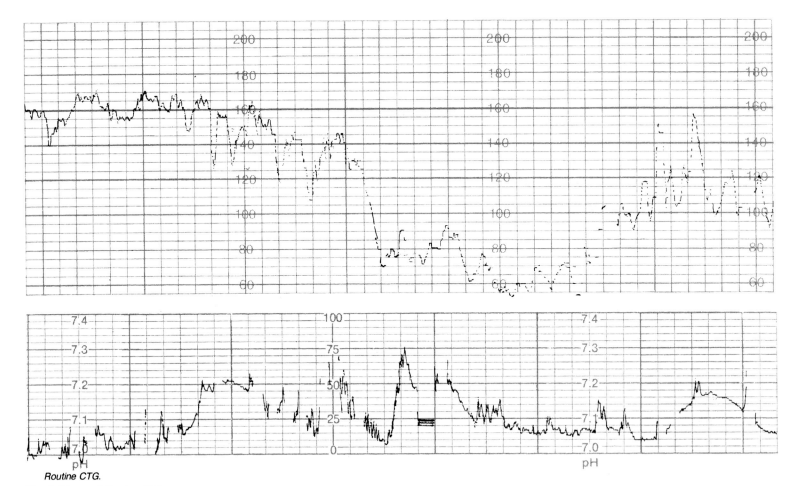

Routine CTG.

Fig. 4.43 *part 1 Routine CTG.*

CTG

1 What do you notice about the baseline?
2 What do you notice about the baseline variability?
3 What periodic changes, if any, are present?
4 What do you notice about the uterine activity?
5 What is the most probable cause of fetal heart rate abnormality shown on this trace?
6 What treatment and/or intervention would you consider necessary for this fetal heart rate pattern?

NOTES

1

2

3

4

5

6

1 Baseline 150–160 b.p.m.
2 Variability external recording, therefore not accurate; appears within normal limits
3 Prolonged deceleration
4 Occasional tightening, no contractions
5 Cord occlusion is a possibility
   Note gestation; placental insufficiency resulting in fetal hypoxia must be considered
6 Prepare for delivery
   Change maternal position
   Give facial oxygen
   Vaginal examination to assess cervix
   If deceleration recovers and cervix favourable, consider surgical induction of labour

15.00 hours
Surgical induction of labour performed
Cervix 1.5 cm long, cervical os 3 cm dilated
Artificial rupture of membranes — fresh meconium-stained liquor draining
Fetal scalp electrode applied
Contractions monitored externally
Contracting spontaneously
15.45 hours
Pethidine 100 mg and Sparine 25 mg given intramuscularly
16.00 hours
CTG — see Part 2, page 220.

CASE STUDY

43

Part 2

OUTCOME [CONTINUED]

16.00 hours
CTG (Fig. 4.43 part 2)

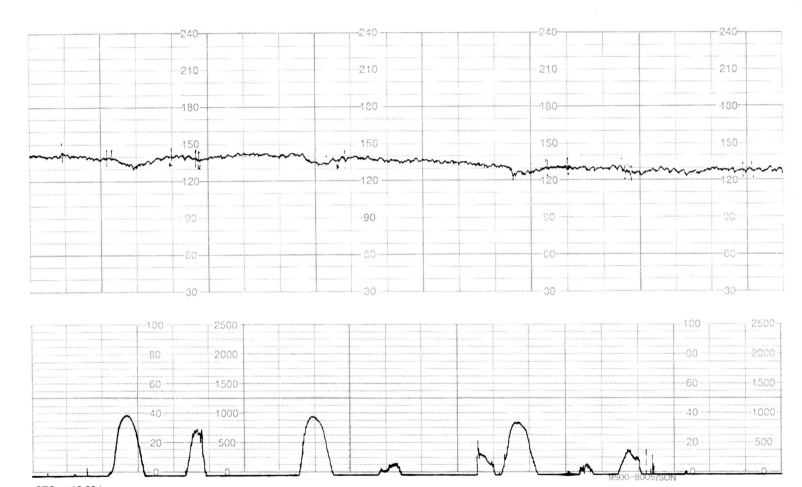

CTG at 16.00 hours.

Fig. 4.43 *part 2 CTG at 16.00 hours.*

CTG

1 What do you notice about the baseline?
2 What do you notice about the baseline variability?
3 What periodic changes, if any, are present?
4 What do you notice about the uterine activity?
5 What is the most probable cause of fetal heart rate abnormality shown on this trace?
6 What treatment and/or intervention would you consider necessary for this fetal heart rate pattern?

NOTES

1

2

3

4

5

6

ANALYSIS

1 Baseline 140–150 b.p.m.
2 Less than 5 b.p.m.
3 Possibly very shallow late decelerations
4 Contracting irregularly, varying in strength; inadequately monitored
5 Pethidine given 15 minutes prior to portion of CTG; however, in view of previous CTG and fresh meconium-stained liquor, fetal hypoxia must be considered
6 Change maternal position
   Give facial oxygen
   Commence intravenous fluids
   Fetal blood sampling is indicated
   If pattern persists, prepare for delivery

OUTCOME

17.00 hours
Cervical os 5 cm dilated
Fetal blood sampling performed: pH 7.20, base excess −10
Caesarean section performed
Live girl
Apgar score 9/1 9/5
Birthweight 4.560 kg
Cord around neck × 1 and around leg × 2

Miscellaneous

HISTORY

20-year-old gravida I, para 0

Past history

Nil relevant

Antenatal period

Normal
Admitted at 40 weeks with contractions

Labour

05.30 hours
Cervical os 5 cm dilated
Artificial rupture of membranes — clear liquor draining
Fetal scalp electrode applied
Intrauterine pressure catheter inserted
06.45 hours
Pethidine 100 mg and Sparine 25 mg given intramuscularly
CTG (Fig. 4.44)

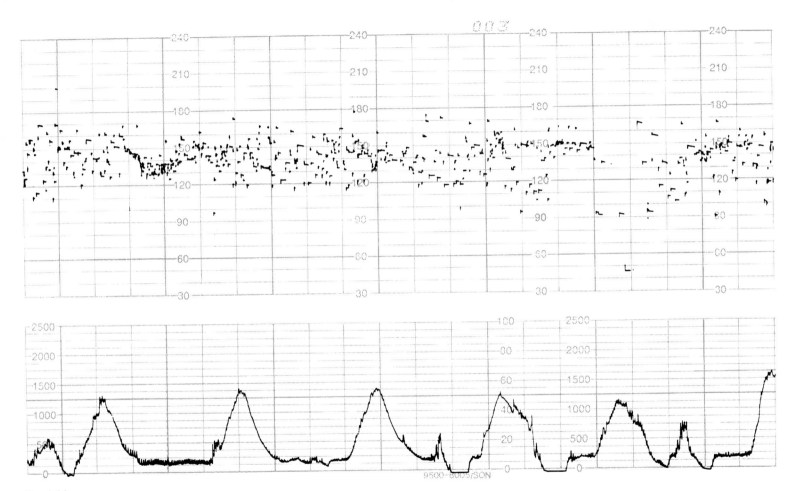

Fig. 4.44

CTG

1 What do you notice about the baseline?
2 What do you notice about the baseline variability?
3 What periodic changes, if any, are present?
4 What do you notice about the uterine activity?
5 What is the most probable cause of fetal heart rate abnormality shown on this trace?
6 What treatment and/or intervention would you consider necessary for this fetal heart rate pattern?

NOTES

1

2

3

4

5

6

ANALYSIS

Impossible to interpret CTG owing to poor quality print-out

6   If fetal scalp electrode not working, monitor externally or use intermittent auscultation. The fetal heart rate should be recorded on the CTG

OUTCOME

13.00 hours
Progressed to second stage of labour
14.25 hours
Spontaneous vertex delivery
Live boy
Apgar score 9/1 9/5
Birthweight 3.250 kg

HISTORY

24-year-old gravida 2, para 1

Past history
Nil relevant

Antenatal period
Normal
Admitted at 40 weeks with spontaneous
rupture of membranes and contractions

Labour
10.30 hours
Cervical os 5 cm dilated
Clear liquor draining
Fetal scalp electrode applied
Contractions monitored externally
Transcutaneous nerve stimulation (TNS) for
analgesia
CTG (Fig. 4.45)

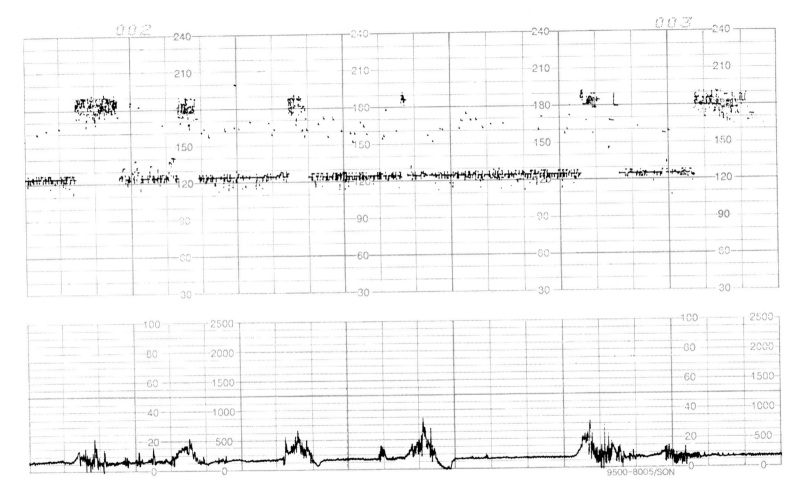

Fig. 4.45

CTG

1 What do you notice about the baseline?
2 What do you notice about the baseline variability?
3 What periodic changes, if any, are present?
4 What do you notice about the uterine activity?
5 What is the most probable cause of fetal heart rate abnormality shown on this trace?
6 What treatment and/or intervention would you consider necessary for this fetal heart rate pattern?

NOTES

1

2

3

4

5

6

ANALYSIS

Impossible to interpret this CTG, owing to electrical interference from TNS

6   Fetal heart should be auscultated and rate written on CTG
    Because of the limited value of the CTG, it is probably better to discontinue it and rely on intermittent auscultation of the fetal heart

OUTCOME

12.30 hours
Second stage of labour diagnosed
12.50 hours
Spontaneous vertex delivery
Live girl
Apgar score 9/1 9/5
Birthweight 3.560 kg

HISTORY

27-year-old gravida 3, para 2

Past history
Nil relevant

Antenatal period
Urinary tract infection treated at 24 weeks' gestation
Normal progress
Admitted at 41 weeks' gestation in spontaneous labour

Labour
13.30 hours
Cervical os 5 cm dilated, membranes intact
Initial CTG normal
15.50 hours
CTG recommenced, external recordings
(Fig. 4.46)

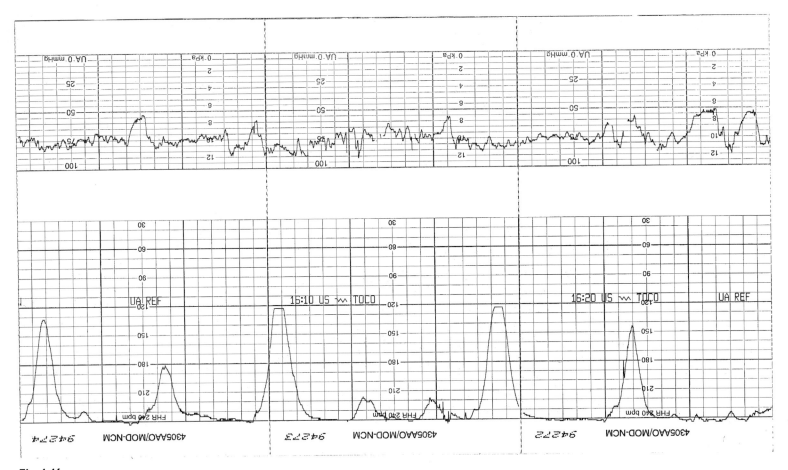

Fig. 4.46

CTG

1 What do you notice about the baseline?
2 What do you notice about the baseline variability?
3 What periodic changes, if any, are present?
4 What do you notice about the uterine activity?
5 What is the most probable cause of fetal heart rate abnormality shown on this trace?
6 What treatment and/or intervention would you consider necessary for this fetal heart rate pattern?

NOTES

1

2

3

4

5

6

1 Baseline, unable to interpret
2 Variability, probably within normal limits
3 Accelerations present, no decelerations
4 Contracting 3 in 10 minutes, varying in strength
5 Probably normal CTG, paper has been loaded into machine upside down
   Despite this the CTG is recorded as being satisfactory in the case notes on two occasions
6 Change paper

Paper rectified after 1 hour
Progressed to normal delivery 3 hours later
Live girl
Apgar score 9/1 9/5
Birthweight 3.380 kg

HISTORY

20-year-old gravida I, para 0

Past history

Nil relevant

Antenatal period

No problems
Admitted at 38 weeks with spontaneous
rupture of membranes and contractions

Labour

13.00 hours
Cervical os 3 cm dilated
Fetal scalp electrode applied
Intrauterine pressure catheter inserted
15.00 hours
No progress, Syntocinon (oxytocin) infusion
commenced
16.30 hours
Epidural analgesia commenced
18.25 hours
Cervical os 6 cm dilated
19.30 hours
Syntocinon (oxytocin) infusing at 10 mU/min
CTG (Fig. 4.47)

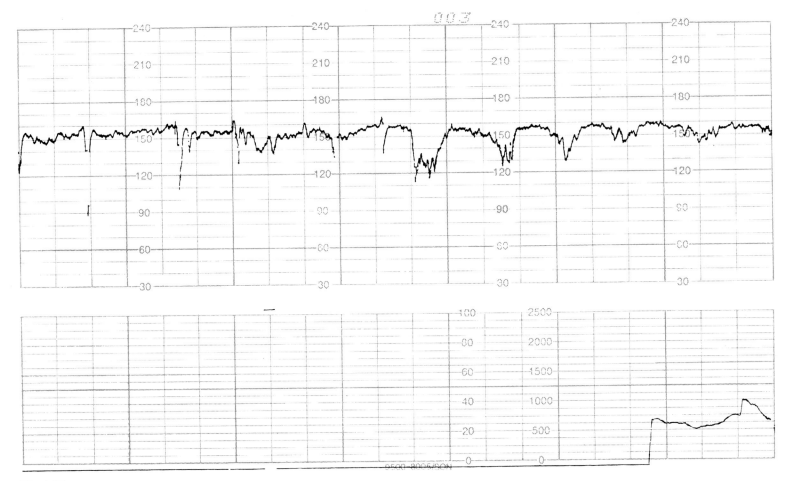

Fig. 4.47

CTG

1 What do you notice about the baseline?
2 What do you notice about the baseline variability?
3 What periodic changes, if any, are present?
4 What do you notice about the uterine activity?
5 What is the most probable cause of fetal heart rate abnormality shown on this chart?
6 What treatment and/or intervention would you consider necessary for this fetal heart rate pattern?

NOTES

1

2

3

4

5

6

ANALYSIS

1 Baseline 150–155 b.p.m.
2 Variability 5 b.p.m.
3 Decelerations cannot be classified as no contractions monitored
4 Contractions not monitored
5 No cause can be attributed
6 Monitor contractions
  Classify decelerations and take appropriate action

OUTCOME

Contractions monitored, decelerations classified as early
20.55 hours
Second stage of labour diagnosed
22.00 hours
Commenced pushing
22.55 hours
Spontaneous vertex delivery
Live girl
Apgar score 9/1 9/5
Birthweight 2.780 kg

48

HISTORY

30-year-old gravida I, para 0

Past history
Nil relevant

Antenatal period
Admitted at 31 weeks with pregnancy-induced hypertension
Admission CTG normal
Blood pressure stabilised
32 weeks
Ultrasound scan shows good growth and normal liquor volume
Routine CTG 2 days later (Fig. 4.48)

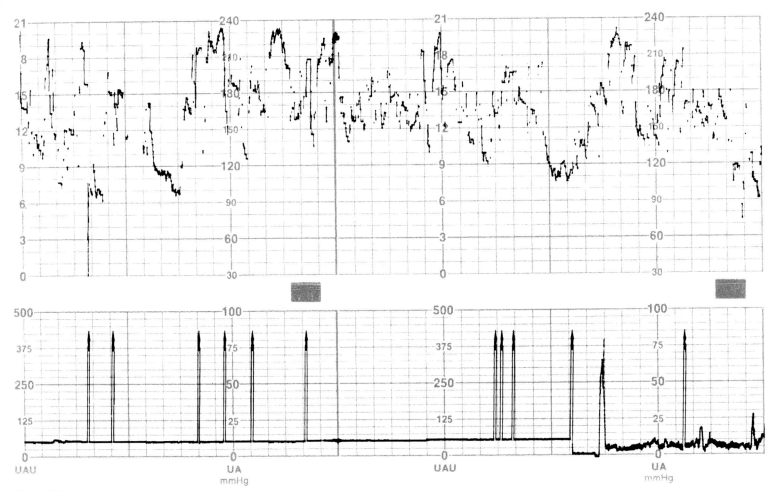

Fig. 4.48 Part I

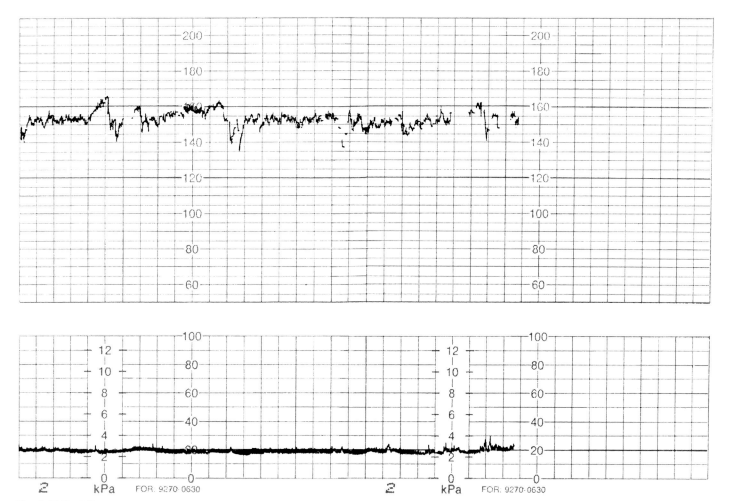

Fig. 4.48 Part 2

CTG

1 What do you notice about the baseline?
2 What do you notice about the baseline variability?
3 What periodic changes, if any, are present?
4 What do you notice about the uterine activity?
5 What is the most probable cause of fetal heart rate abnormality shown on this trace?
6 What treatment and/or intervention would you consider necessary for this fetal heart rate pattern?

NOTES

1

2

3

4

5

6

Impossible to interpret this CTG
6   Fetal heart sounded irregular
      Repeat CTG — similar pattern

Ultrasound scan performed
Structurally normal heart — atrial flutter
diagnosed
Cardiology opinion sought
Mother digitalised
Following day — ultrasound scan shows fetal
heart in normal sinus rhythm
CTG repeated 2 days later — see following
trace
35 weeks
Blood pressure unstable
Caesarean section performed
Live girl
Apgar score 4/1 9/5
Birthweight 1.810 kg
Baby discharged at 3 weeks old — no problems

HISTORY

29-year-old gravida 3, para 2

Past history

Nil of note

Antenatal period

Normal
Admitted in spontaneous labour at 40 weeks gestation

Labour

06.30 hrs
Vaginal assessment revealed the cervix to be thin and well applied to
 presenting part, the cervical os was 4 cm dilated. No analgesia was in use
CTG (Fig. 4.49)

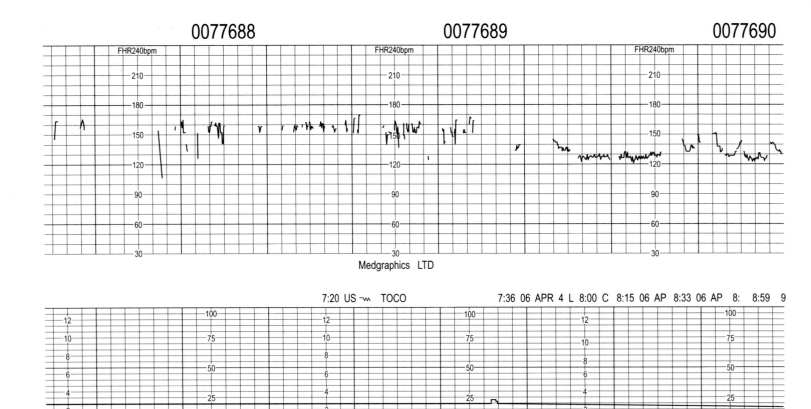

Fig. 4.49

CTG

1 What do you notice about the baseline?
2 What do you notice about the baseline variability?
3 What periodic changes, if any, are present?
4 What do you notice about the uterine activity?
5 What is the most probable cause of fetal heart rate abnormality shown on this trace?
6 What treatment and/or intervention would you consider necessary for this fetal heart rate pattern?

NOTES

1

2

3

4

5

6

ANALYSIS

1 Baseline difficult to decide due to poor contact, possibly 130 b.p.m.
2 Variability, again poor contact makes this difficult, possibly 5 beats
3 Possibly no decelerations with some acceleration
4 Contractions not monitored
5 Could be normal, insufficient data to make a safe judgement
6 Ensure good contact, monitor contractions. This woman was deemed to be low risk for labour; the reason for the CTG should be questioned. Intermittent auscultation should be offered as the preferred method of monitoring the fetal heart rate in labour. If the woman chooses to have continuous monitoring then the risks and benefits as explained to her must be documented in the case notes and her informed consent gained

OUTCOME

Labour progressed well and a live boy was born 2 hours later
Apgar score 9 and 9
In fact intermittent auscultation had been used throughout this labour.
The CTG monitor had been used when auscultating the fetal heart and recorded each time it was listened to, note the times pre printed on the paper. This gives the impression of a continuous CTG. When performing intermittent auscultation the fetal heart rate must be counted for a full minute, and that number documented in the case notes. There should be no recording as this may lead to someone wrongly interpreting the data and potentially instigating unnecessary interventions
Birthweight 3.860 kg

PART 5

Good
Practice guide

Childbirth is a natural process for most women, however for some that process may be interrupted and deviates from normal putting them and their unborn baby at risk. Midwives and obstetricians by the nature of their work become experienced in detecting when all is not well. The correct interpretation of the CTG, based on adequate knowledge of physiology, and the instigation of appropriate management is vital in ensuring that women and their babies are placed at as small a risk as possible of harm due to negligence.

All professionals are responsible for ensuring that they remain updated in all aspects of clinical care, including the interpretation of CTGs, and together with their colleagues should make adequate provision for training and maintaining expertise within their employing Trust.

It is hoped that this practical guide will assist practitioners to access information they may find beneficial and to highlight some areas of good practice that can be shared and disseminated.

DEVELOPING GUIDELINES

Government initiatives have prompted the development of evidence-based guidelines for assessing fetal well being in labour (NICE 2001) and Clinical risk management standards for maternity services (NHS Litigation Authority 2004). However, each Trust has responsibility to ensure that this guidance is incorporated into local guidelines and policies.

These guidelines should be developed by a multi-disciplinary team, be evidence based, clear, easily understood and accessible to all members of staff. It is essential that they are reviewed regularly and updated without delay if necessary. Ideally doctors and midwives should have their own individual copy as well as them being available in each delivery room and area where women in labour, including the latent phase, are cared for. Any revisions made must be communicated to all those with copies of the guidelines.

AUDIT

Audit of clinical practice is an essential component of the quality cycle. Standards and guidelines relating to assessment of fetal well being in labour should be audited regularly to ensure that clinical practice continues to be in line with up-to-date evidence and that current practice equates with good clinical outcomes.

The findings and recommendations from completed audits must be disseminated to all staff. It is also important that any actions are followed through, with key staff members identified to instigate these.

COMMUNICATION

Regular, constructive, multidisciplinary discussions relating to the interpretation and management of CTG abnormalities have been advocated (NHS Litigation Authority 2004, NICE 2001, CESDI 2000). Meetings should be well advertised, convenient for all groups of staff and conducted in a non-threatening manner. Attendance should be documented and form a part of the individuals personal development plan. Practitioners should also be encouraged to discuss the interpretation of CTGs when caring for women in labour. The senior midwife or obstetrician responsible for the department should ensure that this takes place at least once during the course of their shift.

SUPERVISORS OF MIDWIVES

Supervisors of midwives are uniquely placed within the maternity services and should have a strong influence on clinical practice within their employing Trusts. They should be represented on all guideline development groups and audit committees and be at the centre of developing and implementing practice changes. Supervisors meet with their supervisees a minimum of once per year. This discussion should include issues relating to fetal monitoring in labour, developments in clinical practice and the maintenance of clinical skills. In particular, with regard to the assessment of

Birmingham Women's Health Care NHS

NHS Trust

📖 **(7) Version 2: Section 9: Labour Second Stage Fetal Heart Auscultation**
   (continue to complete the partogram documentation for all other observations)

DATE:..

NB: This is NOT intended to be used as a linear scale

To be auscultated after every contraction for a minimum of 1 minute (auscultation should be undertaken a minimum of every 5 minutes)

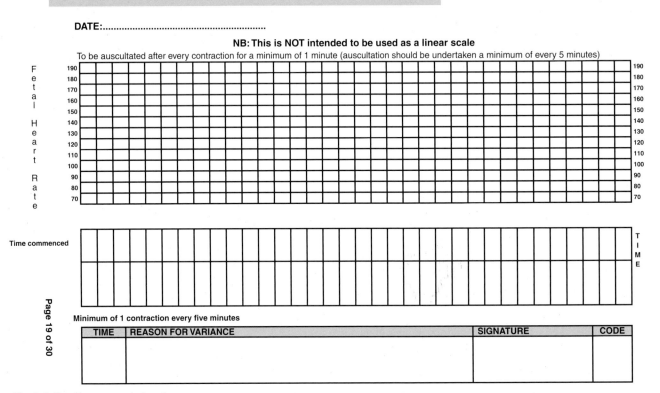

Fetal Heart Rate — 190, 180, 170, 160, 150, 140, 130, 120, 110, 100, 90, 80, 70

Time commenced

TIME

Minimum of 1 contraction every five minutes

TIME	REASON FOR VARIANCE	SIGNATURE	CODE

Fig. 5.1 *Fetal heart ausculation chart.*

Page 19 of 30

fetal well being, use of the Pinard stethoscope should be encouraged. Drop-in sessions and workshops run by Supervisors, in addition to the one-to-one meetings, allow for discussion and should be open to all staff.

PRACTICAL GUIDES

There are occasions when tools can be developed which prove beneficial to clinical practice. Two such tools will be highlighted here, both are in use at Birmingham Women's Health Care NHS Trust, and have been replicated here with permission.

Fetal Heart Auscultation Chart
(Fig. 5.1)
This chart has been designed to be used during the second stage of labour in an attempt to make the documentation easier for the midwife. The chart is incorporated into the labour record following delivery.

CTG Interpretation Stamp (Fig. 5.2). This stamp is used in the case notes and labour record at defined intervals when reviewing the CTG. The purpose is to ensure that important information is documented and that all practitioners use the same criteria for interpretation of the CTG. It is not only the

interpretation that is important, it is also necessary to make a plan for future management dependant upon that interpretation. There is space here to document this. It is good practice to get into the habit of planning any action, even if this is to continue as things are, as it demonstrates that further management has been thought about.

RISK ASSESSMENT CHART

To minimise the risk of untoward occurrences/outcomes, the checklist in

---

C.T.G. REVIEW

Indication for C.T.G. _____

Date: _____ Time: _____

F.H. Baseline: _____ bpm _____

Variability: <5 /5-10 /> 10/ bpm

Accelerations: Yes / No

Decelerations: Yes / No Define _____

Action: _____

Name: _____ Signature: _____

C.T.G. REVIEW

Indication for C.T.G. _____

Date: _____ Time: _____

F.H. Baseline: _____ bpm _____

Variability: <5 /5-10 /> 10/ bpm

Accelerations: Yes / No

Decelerations: Yes / No Define _____

Action: _____

Name: _____ Signature: _____

Fig. 5.2 *CTG interpretation stamp.*

Table 5.1 Checklist of questions

	Yes	No
Are you confident and competent in the interpretation of the CTG?	❏	❏
Have you been trained and are you familiar with all the fetal monitoring equipment used in the clinical setting in which you work?	❏	❏
Are you aware of the facilities and personnel available for the repair and maintenance of equipment?	❏	❏
Are you satisfied with your knowledge of the research evidence, with regard to fetal monitoring, and do you base your practice upon this?	❏	❏
Are you comfortable in communicating any concerns regarding the interpretation of a CTG?	❏	❏
Do you obtain consent (informed) from women prior to commencing continuous fetal monitoring?	❏	❏
Do you attend regular multidisciplinary updating and training events in the interpretation of CTGs?	❏	❏
Is your record-keeping maintained to the highest standard; is it clear, concise, legible and unambiguous?	❏	❏
When making records relating to a CTG, in the case notes, do you describe the baseline, variability, reactivity and presence or absence of any decelerations as opposed to writing 'normal' or 'satisfactory'?	❏	❏
Is there a means of storing CTGs within the case notes that ensures that they do not get lost?	❏	❏

Table 5.1 has been compiled in relation to cardiotocography and should be used in conjunction with your employer's policies, protocols or guidelines and any rules, codes of practice and guidelines concerning the framework within which you practise as a doctor or midwife. For midwives, these will be those set out by the Nursing and Midwifery Council (NMC). For doctors they will be those of the employer.

Both groups must be familiar with any guidelines and/or protocols set out by an NHS trust or other place of work outside the NHS. This should also include advice and standards set by other recognised national bodies.

If the answer to any of the questions in Table 5.1 is 'No', then ask yourself 'What must I do about it?' Is it a matter for you, your colleagues, your supervisor of midwives, your manager?

The NMC distributes the documents specified in Table 5.2 to all practitioners on the register. They are revised from time to time and it is the responsibility of each midwife to be familiar with their contents and refer to them as and when appropriate. If you do not have copies of any of the NMC documents on the list, then write to the NMC at: 23 Portland Place, London, W1N 4JT.

Do you have a copy of the most up to date publications relevant to your practice, and are you familiar with their contents?

Midwives Rules and Standards	2004
Code of Professional Conduct	2002
Guidelines for records and record keeping	2002

Are you familiar with all documents relating to areas of your practice?

Trust standards and guidelines
Royal College of Obstetricians and Gynaecologists advice and guidance
Nursing and Midwifery advice and guidance
The National Institute for Clinical Excellence guidelines
Clinical Negligence Scheme for Trusts standards
Local Supervising Authority (LSA) for midwives standards.

Excellent communication is essential when developing good practice guides. This includes discussions with colleagues within the same unit and with those from other Trusts. Sharing of information is vital and benchmarking practice and outcomes with other comparable units should be commonplace. Practitioners

Table 5.2 Checklist of documents relating to practice

	Yes	No
Do you have a copy of the most up-to-date publications relevant to your practice, and are you familiar with their contents?	❏	❏
Midwives' Rules and Standards 2004	❏	❏
Code of Professional Conduct 2002	❏	❏
Guidelines for records and record keeping 2002	❏	❏
Are you familiar with all documents relating to areas of your practice?	❏	❏
Trust standards and guidelines	❏	❏
Royal College of Obstetricians and Gynaecologists advice and guidance	❏	❏
Nursing and Midwifery advice and guidance	❏	❏
The National Institute for Clinical Excellence guidelines	❏	❏
Clinical Negligence Scheme for Trusts standards	❏	❏
Local Supervising Authority (LSA) for midwives' standards	❏	❏

who have been involved in the planning and implementation of good practice initiatives must be encouraged to write about their experiences and the benefits that can be demonstrated. Publishing of such work in professional journals will then provide the forum for dissemination of information and discussion.

Ultimately we practise within our professions in order to provide care for women and babies that will ensure they are as free from risk as possible. Happy, healthy families are the main aim, each individual practitioner has a duty to ensure that their practise does not hinder this.

WEB ADDRESSES

There are a large number of web sites that can be easily accessed that are useful when searching for information. Some of these are listed below and most of them will have links to other sites. Many medical and midwifery journals are now available on line, free of charge.

Department of Health www.doh.gov.uk
NICE www.nice.org.uk
Royal College of Obstetricians and Gynaecologists www.rcog.org.uk
Nursing and Midwifery Council www.nmc-uk.org
Confidential enquiry into maternal and child health www.cemach.org.uk
Association for Improvements in Maternity Services www.aims.org.uk

REFERENCES

CESDI (2000) 7th Annual report. Maternal and Child health Research Consortium, London
NICE (2001) The use of electronic fetal monitoring. Inherited clinical guideline C. NICE, London
NHS Litigation Authority (2004) Clinical negligence scheme for trusts. Clinical risk management standards for the maternity services. NHS Litigation Authority, London

INDEX